Innovations in Professional Education for Speech and Language Therapy

Innovations in Professional Education for Speech and Language Therapy

Edited by

Shelagh Brumfitt PhD, MPhil, RegMRCSLT, MHPC
Department of Human Communication Sciences
University of Sheffield

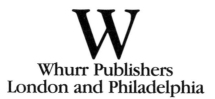

Whurr Publishers
London and Philadelphia

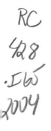
British Library Cataloguing in Publication Data

A catalogue record for this book is available from the British Library.

ISBN 1 86156 385 X

Typeset by Adrian McLaughlin, a@microguides.net
Printed and bound in the UK
by Athenæum Press Ltd, Gateshead, Tyne & Wear.

Contents

Foreword

Shelagh Brumfitt, in the introduction to this book, describes the necessity for and purpose of this text. She also outlines the main themes and directions of each section, so what is left to write is a 'Foreword'. May I fall back on the personal perspective of a clinician, speech and language therapy researcher and service manager who has strayed into the world of academia and education.

As a student many years ago, faced with learning primarily through the 'being lectured at' mode, I, along with many others, lost interest and enthusiasm. In my case, this interest and enthusiasm was rekindled by some productive placements, dampened by other placements, but reignited by my first job, where I quickly learned the difficulty of applying remote theory to demanding, immediate practice, much of which seemed to be unrelated to anything in any flow diagram.

The emphasis on ensuring that gained knowledge can be used in different ways to address new problems and applications is a theme running through this book. There are no health or social care professions that I know of where all the fundamental knowledge is unquestioned and can be learned as a 'truth' to be applied in a prescribed and unrefutable manner.

While each discipline does have core elements, principles and facts, there remains a great deal which relies on bringing knowledge together in unique combinations to contribute to a unique situation. Evidence-based care and guidelines to all clinical practice will probably only ever give the defined and tested procedures for less than 20% of any human care process. While it is essential that students are 'taught' these 'truths', it is equally essential that they know how to proceed with the myriad of unusual issues that need to be addressed on a daily basis in every clinic.

As a therapist and manager, I found it hard to understand why students were not 'taught how to treat'. It is only with passing years that one realizes that this would be an impossible ambition and that learning how to identify and solve a range of clinical problems is a basic skill that is transferable and generalizable, thus equipping the student to develop competency beyond that of a checklist of skills attained.

There was a time when academia had an abreaction to the term 'application', seeing this as an avenue that would lead to corruption of academic purity where theories developed, argued and defended within the mind were unsullied by practical considerations and demonstrable exceptions. Fortunately, as several chapters in this book demonstrate, the practical clinical world is now recognized as a rich learning resource, as long as it is incorporated appropriately rather than it being a place to plant students who may fortuitously learn something of value. The divide between the university department and the workplace is less stark, with an appreciation that clinicians are now more involved with the education of students, and university departments recognizing that education and curriculum development must incorporate an employer perspective and lead to student experience that will result in a clinician who is 'fit to practise'.

It is interesting that all of the chapters within this book draw on literature and experience related to the education of other healthcare professions. These chapters will also contribute to the education of students in professions other than speech and language therapy. The interprofessional learning agenda has grown from the recognition that all health professions share some core philosophies, principles, skills and attitudes, and while each requires its own specific unique knowledge there will be gains if commonalities are also recognized and respected.

One of the issues not addressed in this book and thus something I feel I can add specifically, rather than simply regurgitating it in this Foreword, is the importance of enthusing the student in his or her chosen topic. A student who develops sufficient belief, as well as knowledge and love for a subject, will continue to learn throughout the course of his or her career.

Pam Enderby
July 2003

Contributors

Sue Baxter has been a practising speech and language therapist for 16 years, with experience of working with a broad range of client groups and service management. She is currently a clinical tutor at the University of Sheffield, where she is responsible for the clinical components of the undergraduate and postgraduate degree courses leading to qualification as a speech and language therapist.

Shelagh Brumfitt is a senior lecturer in the Department of Human Communication Sciences at the University of Sheffield. She is the programme director for the undergraduate qualifying course in speech and language therapy, and chair of the departmental clinical education research group.

Richard Cox is a reader in the School of Cognitive and Computing Sciences at the University of Sussex. He studied psychology and education before doing a PhD in artificial intelligence at the University of Edinburgh. He is a cognitive scientist whose interests include interactive learning environments, human reasoning and individual differences.

Barbara Dodd has worked in paediatric speech and language therapy since 1968, working in clinical and academic departments of linguistics, psychology and speech in the UK and Australia. She is currently Professor of Speech and Language Therapy in the Speech and Language Sciences programme at University of Newcastle. She has been involved in setting up problem-based learning courses at Queensland University, University of Newcastle, UK, and Trinity College, Dublin. Her research interests are in phonological acquisition and disorders.

Sue Franklin is currently senior lecturer on the Speech and Language Sciences programme at University of Newcastle, UK. Her key research activity has been the analysis and treatment of aphasia, with a particular interest in evaluating intensive therapy in a large group study in

Newcastle. Her interests extend also to phonological and sentence processing impairments in aphasia, comparison of developmental and acquired phonological disorders and the development of psycholinguistic assessments in Japanese aphasia.

Margaret Freeman is a lecturer in speech and language therapy in the Department of Human Communication Sciences at the University of Sheffield. She has a special interest in promoting the use of information and communication technologies for clinical work, teaching and research, and has recently completed an MEd in e-learning.

Kim Grundy is principal lecturer in speech and language therapy at De Montfort University, Leicester. She was programme leader and clinical placements co-ordinator for the speech and language therapy degree programme from 1993 to 2001. During this time, she developed a model of peer placements and peer-tutoring placements which is now an integral part of the clinical practice placement programme. She is a registered homeopath, and divides her time between teaching personal and professional development and her homeopathic practice.

Kirsten Hoben qualified as a speech and language therapist in 1989 and has practised for the past 13 years, mostly in the NHS. From September 2000 to December 2001 she worked as project assistant on the NMET-funded study 'Informing Educational Change to Improve the Professional Competence of Speech and Language Therapists'.

Carmel Lum is a qualified speech and language therapist and chartered psychologist. She began her career in Australia in neuro-rehabilitation before receiving further degree qualifications in research methods and a PhD in cognitive neuropsychology at York. Her interest in clinical reasoning in students and experts grew out of her experiences as a lecturer in aphasiology and research methods. She is currently a Senior Research Fellow at the Human Communication Research Centre, University of Edinburgh.

Sue Pownall works as a specialist speech and language therapist in the clinical area of dysphagia in Sheffield. She is a course leader and lecturer for the basic-level Sheffield dysphagia course, which is credit rated to masters level at Sheffield Hallam University, and is currently managing a project implementing partnership working between the speech and language therapy and nursing professions in the assessment and management of dysphagia.

Jois Stansfield is a qualified speech and language therapist and is head of speech and language sciences at Queen Margaret University College, Edinburgh. She worked in a number of posts in England and Canada before moving to Scotland to specialise in clinical work with learning disability and dysfluency. Her current post involves research and teaching and she maintains a clinical commitment in the Scottish Centre for Speech Disability. Her most recent research work has focused on the clinical education of pre-qualifying speech and language therapy students and the development of competence for entry into the profession.

Anne Whitworth has worked in both Australia and the UK, her clinical work spanning both adult and child communication disorders. She is currently Director of Clinical Education on the Speech and Language Sciences programme at University of Newcastle, UK, where clinical education of speech and language therapists is a key area of interest. Other research interests are the evaluation of treatment efficacy in aphasia and the development of sound clinical assessment measures, particularly in elucidating sentence processing disorders and in applying conversation analysis to the assessment process.

Acknowledgements

I would like to thank Professor Joy Stackhouse, Department of Human Communication Sciences, University of Sheffield, for the original conversation which created the idea for this book. Secondly, I would like to thank all contributing authors for their goodwill and co-operation in completing the work.

Introduction
Perspectives in professional education, an overview

SHELAGH BRUMFITT

During the development of speech and language therapy as a profession, several core texts have been written about professional education as a specific subject (Stengelhofen, 1993; McAllister et al., 1997). Each of these texts has marked a milestone in the evolution of the subject of teaching clinical skills relevant to the speech and language therapy context. Yet, compared to the vast number of textbooks written on theoretical aspects of communication impairment, the number of professional education texts is extremely small. There is clearly an important lesson to learn about how a profession develops. An example of this can be seen in medical education, which reflects the same pattern: the development of a substantial knowledge base about disease without a parallel framework for the process of teaching about disease. In medicine, the knowledge about teaching clinical education has grown only relatively recently (Newble and Entwistle, 1986; Newble and Cannon, 1994).

Within the last decade, as with medicine, there has been an increased interest in the ways in which an individual comes to have the appropriate knowledge and skills to function as a qualified speech and language therapist. As a professional subject, speech and language therapy has developed substantially, drawing on other academic areas to bring together the complete discipline. Linguistics, psychology and biomedical sciences have formed the basis of the epistemology from which clinical application has been derived, but this has been a complex route to the unified subject of speech and language therapy. During this process, the profession has been teaching its students to learn academic and professional material in a higher education context. However, although the purer academic aspects of the degree can be taught from within the institution, higher education can only serve the needs of these students if the professional experience modules are met from outside. Professional education is a notably different process from that of higher education for a theoretical degree, and although the institution can provide teaching in professional methods, the application has to be found within the actual work context. This is what makes teaching a qualifying course in speech and language therapy so administratively complex. Yet, in spite of the huge challenges professional education brings, 'there has been comparatively little written about professional education as a field of study distinct from higher education' (Taylor, 1997: 3).

We now recognize that the professional education we provide for our students critically influences how well prepared they are for the workplace. In the special case of professional subjects, the primary objective is to prepare the student for professional practice, which is of critical importance for the clients awaiting help.

A range of educational frameworks exists to take the student through the various stages of academic and professional development. Providing education that covers both theoretical understanding and practical experience clearly needs differing educational contexts. Many years ago, Polanyi (1958) recognized the major distinction to be made between explicit and tacit knowledge. Explicit knowledge is about the objective, public, theory-driven knowledge that students bring to the clinical setting, whereas tacit knowledge is knowing about the professional role, based on experience. How that has been taken forward in many professions has been a cause for concern, with recognition that the explicit knowledge may have, in the past, been given more emphasis than the tacit.

Preparing to be 'oven ready'? (*The Times*, 2002)

In a recently reported speech, the chair of the Committee of Vice Chancellors and Principals (CVCP) described graduates of higher education as needing to be 'oven ready' in order to be prepared for the challenges of the workplace. Although some of this referred to the need for graduates to have transferable skills, it is easy to see its relevance to those entering the healthcare professions. The assumption is that the newly qualified therapist can move smoothly into competent practice, the preparation having all been done beforehand.

Until recently, traditional universities have held on to the belief that the lecture is still the most effective way of teaching students. This has its basis in a long history. Brown and Atkins (1990) discuss the development of lecturing from the fifth century BC. In medieval times, the lecture is reported as being used at both Christian and Muslim universities and the process of reading a text out loud was established at that time. Although lecturing technique has developed since then, the concept that lecturing is the best way to enable students to understand difficult concepts is still very much with us. Indeed, the lecture can provide students with frameworks for understanding new concepts in all aspects of the course, but it is how the student makes the application from knowledge and understanding to therapeutic skills and attitudes which is critical in a professional degree. Integrating theory and practice on university-based courses with the professional experiences on placement can be difficult.

So, how can we help our own students to understand the complete process of professional activity? We know that lecturing does not provide the means for students to have a deep understanding of the work-based context. As a response to this we have developed other approaches to teaching, which are reflected in the educational techniques used today. All speech and language therapy qualifying courses now include a mix of lecture-based teaching, workshops, tutorials and seminars on the university site, along with the learning and teaching acquired in the clinical placement. A spiral curriculum is often used in order to return several times to the same material, with increasing demands on the student in terms of complexity. Yet, as Bines (1992) notes, although professional education is central to the degree, it has proved to be the least well-developed element of most courses. Although it is a formalized experience, the amount of structure in speech and language therapy clinical placements has been slow to increase and often this is difficult to control because the work context can be a very unpredictable setting. The placement can be influenced by variations in client behaviours, changes to educational and healthcare routines, the general unpredictability of working in an environment where one telephone call can change the activities for a session – in fact, a myriad of unexpected factors. Originally, an apprenticeship model was used for the student therapist on placement. We can be pleased that our professional learning has now moved on to a model of an active learner who participates in all aspects of the placement context.

But what does the process involve? Professional learning on placements is not small group teaching, neither is it just shadowing a professional (unless that is the purpose of the placement). Professional learning has to be able to provide the student with a developing set of skills and understanding to be able to finally achieve clinical competence. It is the key to the main purpose of the degree and provides the opportunity for all of the contributing disciplines to integrate. As McAllister et al. (1997: 6) state, 'Clinical education is about the real world of professional practice where learning is holistic and involves transfer, reorganisation, application, synthesis and evaluation of previously acquired knowledge.'

Eraut (1992) described the three strands which contribute to the kind of knowledge essential for professional education. These have remained a useful framework for understanding what we do. First, Eraut describes propositional knowledge, that of the general principles and discipline-based concepts which form the core understanding of the qualification and the determinants of professional action. Second, personal knowledge and the interpretation of experience form the second strand. Eraut emphasizes the importance of this aspect in professions where interpersonal skill is essential, although enabling personal knowledge to be used in the development of a professional may have to be facilitated. Finally, process knowledge is defined and refers to the knowledge about how to conduct the processes involved in professional activity. Eraut defined five types of process involved in this:

- acquiring information – how the individual selects and implements methods of enquiry
- skilled behaviour – the acquisition of routine behaviours in professional practice
- deliberative processes – involving planning, decision making and problem solving
- giving information – which includes being able to work out what is needed
- controlling one's own behaviour – using self-knowledge and self-management to do so.

As Taylor (1997) comments, different professions will vary in what emphasis they put on these different aspects, but clearly the use of personal and process knowledge has to be influential in developing the role of the speech and language therapist.

What is in the book?

All the subsequent chapters in this book attest to the major developments that are taking place in professional education, not only in an increase of the knowledge base but also an increase in the skill base.

The book includes material from clinical educators at many of the UK speech and language therapy qualifying courses and from speech and language therapists in service delivery. It represents the current issues and initiatives in professional education and reveals a broad base, drawing on expertise from specific subject areas, to wider aspects of higher education learning and teaching.

Each chapter has been written to stand alone. Although they are grouped into themed sections, they can be read in any order. All of them address aspects of professional education which have needed further consideration and for which there is little already written. Each chapter sets out its own theoretical framework. The book also responds to changes in the client's context; that is, recent developments in the educational setting, the NHS setting and in information technology. The themed sections are summarized below.

Aspects of the process

In the first chapter, we are introduced to the concept of competence for speech and language therapy practice. As with many of the terms used in speech and language therapy education, competence is frequently used as a general descriptor, but this chapter examines the theoretical under-pinning of the concept of competence and relates it to the speech and language therapy context. As will be evident from this, competence is nei-ther unidimensional nor a universally agreed concept, but it takes us through the various models of competence which are giving us a better understanding of what it is a speech and language therapy student has to be able to demonstrate to achieve a satisfactory standard. In addition, Jois Stansfield provides us with a summary of work completed on asking stu-dents, qualified speech and language therapists, and educators about their perceptions of how competence is constructed.

One development in the area of professional and clinical education relates to that of the problem-based learning approach. In Chapter 2, we are introduced to the implementation of this approach at the University of Newcastle. Problem-based learning approaches are well developed in other professional areas and an example of this is medicine, where this is still somewhat controversial. Educators have to be able to reconceptualize the model of traditional education, which was a series of sequential courses giving the student theoretical knowledge before clinical knowl-edge. As has been demonstrated in medicine, providing the student with a problem-based approach, where learning is based around clinical/profes-sional problems, allows students to be confronted with real-life contexts immediately. This approach is based in learning theories which have shown that knowledge is memorized and understood more efficiently if it originates in a context that is going to be used and relevant in the future (Newble and Cannon, 1994). Anne Whitworth, Sue Franklin and Barbara Dodd provide an overview of the development of problem-based learning and discuss the rationale for delivering this in the speech and language therapy degree. An outline of the teaching process is provided, with exam-ples of how it is organized in the educational setting. Evaluation of this approach is also discussed. Many speech and language therapy courses in the UK are turning to this approach, and this chapter provides a lead in this area.

In Chapter 3, Kim Grundy discusses the use of peer placements in the professional educational setting. This chapter focuses on an evaluation of this approach with a discussion of its theoretical framework. Unlike many other professional learning contexts, speech and language therapists have provided clinical teaching in a setting which is usually one to one. Peer placements, which have been shown to provide a quality learning envi-ronment, are seen as innovations in this context. Grundy provides practical material to encourage the reader new to this approach and addresses many of the potential advantages and disadvantages.

Shelagh Brumfitt and Kirsten Hoben examine a different aspect of professional education in Chapter 4; that of the transition from university to the workplace on qualification. Professional socialization has been discussed widely, but often not looked at in the context of other professional groups. Here, the literature from many different professionals such as teachers, doctors and social workers is used to highlight the issues which face the newly qualified therapist. Major themes from a study of speech and language therapy managers and newly qualified therapists identify areas of concern which need further research. Although this is an area that needs more investigation, the commonalities between the transitional developments in speech and language therapy and other professions are striking.

Specific educational contexts

In the subject-specific section of the book, two chapters look at the health and educational context in order to examine approaches to teaching and learning. To a certain extent, the professional learning experience has been related to the type of placement or the topic as it occurs within the degree syllabus. What these two chapters show is how the nature of the professional activity is now influencing the content and organization of the teaching. Dysphagia is a specific example of the profession taking on this new discipline, so that qualifying courses have had to respond to the requirements of the workplace in precise ways to meet the needs of the clients.

In Chapter 5, Sue Pownall has written one of the first discussions on the approach to the teaching of dysphagia. As many readers will know, the compulsory requirement for basic-level competency in dysphagia has meant that university courses are now required to incorporate this into their degree programme. However, although there is a well-developed structure for post-qualification levels, this has been less developed at the pre-qualification level. Competency standards are discussed with reference to the Royal College of Speech and Language Therapists, American Speech and Hearing Association and Speech Pathology; Australia. Specific guidelines are given about methods for teaching this area, with a discussion on ethics in this context. What is of particular interest here is that the standards for dysphagia clinical teaching have been worked out in much more detail than other communication impairment areas. Future developments may need to include competencies in each diagnostic category.

Sue Baxter's evaluation of the placement-based learning in Chapter 6 provides a model for designing innovative clinical placements. The chapter discusses traditional approaches to placements and builds on this model to show how new ways of working with students and with the actual work contexts can bring about a modernized education. Each of three types of placements (mainstream school, nursery and acute hospital) is described with a discussion of the ways in which the students were organized and provided with active learning experiences. It is demonstrated that requiring students to take more responsibility for their own learning and practice, enables them to mature and give something back to the work placement.

Information technology: developments and applications

The progress in information technology has provided the educational setting with a series of exciting opportunities for enabling students' professional understanding. In Chapter 7, Margaret Freeman gives an overview of the ways in which this can be used, with an evaluation of different aspects of the work. Students can make use of the World Wide Web, computer simulations, computer-assisted learning, e-learning and networked learning, all of which provide evidence for the huge educational changes made in the last decade. The chapter gives examples of ways to apply these technologies, with guidance on how to help students gain expertise with different approaches.

In Chapter 8, Richard Cox and Carmel Lum describe their specialized innovation – PATSy, a web-based multimedia system which provides students with 'virtual' patients and opportunities for case-based learning and clinical reasoning tasks (developed at Queen Margaret University College and Edinburgh University). For those in the higher education setting, having a resource where students can practise before coming face to face with 'live' clients can be exceptionally advantageous. This chapter addresses the theoretical rationale for the development of PATSy, with a description of how it may be used. In addition, its use in understanding clinical reasoning skills is reported.

Who is this book for?

We all know what it is like to be a student and to learn how to become a professional; learning eventually what enables or disables that process. This book is for the reader who is aware of the complicated path to qualification, who can appreciate the challenges and demands and who has responsibility for ensuring others learn the appropriate skills.

All the professional academic staff who work in university departments on speech and language therapy courses may find the material in this book stimulating. In addition, those clinical teachers who are in the work context of schools, hospitals and communities will find information and understanding to further their own skill base. Others from related healthcare or education-based professions may find the material applicable to their own area. Many of the approaches here have been influenced by other professional practices and there are clearly common interests.

References

Bines H (1992) Issues in course design. In Bines H, Watson D (eds) Developing Professional Education. Buckingham: Open University Press.

Brown G, Atkins M (1990) Effective Teaching in Higher Education. London: Routledge.

Eraut M (1992) Developing the professional knowledge base: a process perspective on professional education. In Barnett R (ed.) Learning to Effect. Buckingham: Society for Research into Higher Education and the Open University Press.

McAllister L, Lincoln M, McLeod S, Maloney D (1997) Facilitating Learning in Clinical Settings. Cheltenham: Stanley Thornes.

Newble D, Cannon R (1994) A Handbook for Medical Teachers, 3rd edn. London: Kluwer Academic Publishers.

Newble DI, Entwistle NJ (1986) Learning styles and approaches: implications for medical education. Medical Education 20: 162–175.

Polanyi M (1958) Personal knowledge. London: Routledge and Kegan Paul.

Stengelhofen J (1993) Teaching Students in Clinical Settings. Cheltenham: Stanley Thornes.

Taylor I (1997) Developing Learning in Professional Education. Buckingham: Society for Research into Higher Education and the Open University Press.

The Times (2002) Who said what? The Times Weekend 6 July.

PART I
ASPECTS OF THE PROCESS

Chapter 1
Education for competent speech and language therapy practice

JOIS STANSFIELD

Introduction

Why do speech and language therapists need to be competent? There are answers at many levels. From a personal point of view, each speech and language therapist might be expected to wish to do the best they can in the interests of their clients and themselves, leading to an enhanced sense of personal worth. Professionally, speech and language therapists have a duty to provide a level of care that is appropriate and sufficient to meet the communicative needs of clients. At a regulatory level, the professional body (the Royal College of Speech and Language Therapists, RCSLT) has a duty to protect the reputation of its members, and the statutory body (the Health Professions Council) has a duty to protect the public. Competent practice is essential if these duties are to be fulfilled, and incompetent practice will be disciplined with the aim of assuring these outcomes.

Competence has many identities, from 'good enough' to 'excellent'. This chapter explores differing approaches to competence and relates them to the speech and language therapy experience of education for practice through a study of the views of three groups of 'stakeholders' involved in speech and language therapy education. Drawn from this, the chapter presents a model of the development of clinical competence in speech and language therapy education. The chapter concludes with a brief discussion of the complex nature of developing competence in speech and language therapy education.

Theories of competence

A fundamental issue in defining competence is that the word is used to represent significantly differing philosophies. At one end of the spectrum, competence is seen on a binary scale: a person either is or is not competent, based on published itemized criteria. At the opposite end are approaches with their roots in concepts of expert practice and educational and philosophical thinking. Here, judgements of competence involve qualitative as well as quantitative aspects. They address capability (identification of potential) as well as evidence of current performance and usually include consideration of the mental processes involved in using knowledge in decision making.

Between these poles are Gonczi's (1994) description of Australian approaches to identifying competence and the attribute-based management school approach to competence exemplified by the McBer organization (Spencer and Spencer, 1993).

The NVQ approach

National (and Scottish) Vocational Qualifications (NVQs) were introduced into the UK as an attempt to provide a coherent single entity for vocational qualifications, rather than the patchwork approach Jessup (1991) suggested was available up to the mid-1980s. NVQs have an outcomes-based assessment system, whereby each element of occupational activity is identified and assessed, and once all elements have been completed successfully the NVQ candidate is certificated as competent.

NVQs are assigned at levels from 1 to 5 and have notional correspondence to educational qualifications (see Table 1.1).

Table 1.1 Notional correspondence of qualifications.

Higher degree	N/SVQ 5
Degrees	
	N/SVQ 4
A level/AS level/ Scottish Higher	N/SVQ 3
	N/SVQ 2
GCSE/Standard Grade	N/SVQ 1

There are major criticisms of the NVQ system in relation to professional competence (e.g. Gonczi, 1994; Hager and Hyland, 2002). First, learning is separated from a syllabus or curriculum. The implication is that the NVQ model, unlike most educational approaches, is not concerned with the process of learning. Second, in the NVQ model all elements of competence are required to be assessed separately, but the system does not allow for an assessment of the overall performance or capability of a candidate. The implication is that the whole of competence, in NVQ terms, is precisely and only the sum of its parts. Third, knowledge is not addressed in a satisfactory manner. The place of knowledge in the NVQ definition of competence is of particular relevance in the consideration of learning at higher levels. Jessup (1991), the main author of the NVQ system, was clear that skill could not exist without (unassessed) underpinning knowledge and understanding required to achieve competent performance. Knowledge itself, however, is not to be assessed directly: the existence of skill is deemed sufficient to prove the existence of knowledge and understanding. NVQs therefore appear unsuited to defining pre-qualifying professional competence.

The Australian approach

At around the same time as the NVQ framework was being developed in the UK, work was taking place in Australia to develop 'competency-based standards' for professional work (Gonczi et al., 1990; Gonczi, 1994). Gonczi et al.'s outline of the competent practitioner is one who has the capacity to use a complex interaction of knowledge, attitudes, values and skills ('attributes' or 'competencies' in his terminology) in a range of contexts. In speech and language therapy for example, the knowledge base would need to mesh with ethical standards and the ability to communicate with clients. Gonczi defines competence as capacity, emphasizing that the judgements of competence must incorporate the 'holistic integrated performances' (1994: 35) in the person's work. Poor performance in one area of competence can be compensated by strengths elsewhere. The emphasis is on the integration of skills and knowledge, with an ability to utilize these appropriately in context.

There is little discussion of this model in the British literature, but it appears to avoid the disadvantages of the NVQ approach (Hager and Hyland, 2002). It takes account of the nature of professional practice, and Australian professions appear to accept the model because they have been involved in its development.

An attributes view of professional competence

A number of business schools in the United States have approached the development and definition of competence from a quite different angle from those outlined above. McBer and colleagues (e.g. Spencer and Spencer, 1993) modelled a system of identifying competence derived from observing expert practitioners, which takes account predominantly of personal attributes rather than on-task performance. Spencer and Spencer talk of 'competency', but define a competency as:

> an underlying characteristic of an individual which is causally related to the criterion-referenced performance in a variety of situations. (1993: 9)

This underlying characteristic is 'a deep and enduring part of the person's personality' (1993: 9) which will predict behaviour in a variety of structures.

The underlying characteristics or competencies Spencer and Spencer specify are the person's motives, traits, self-concept, knowledge and skill. In their definition, motives, traits and self-concept 'competencies' produce skill, and skill predicts outcomes. The competencies are, however, deeply buried and, being central to the personality, they are far more difficult to develop or measure than knowledge or skills.

Some notes of caution are needed in considering this approach. The entire system is culturally embedded in the US and, specifically, has been devised in business schools. Much of the work appears to assume that there is one particular type of 'good' worker in any given field and there are some dated stereotypes in the clusters of traits claimed to be necessary, at least for the fields of education and healthcare. To an extent, the argument appears to be not one of educating but of recruiting the right people in the first place, begging the question: is the competent worker born or made? If traits *are* taken to be central, those which are proposed to be typical of superior performers appear largely to be within a masculine frame of behaviour, a fact acknowledged in later work by the same research group (Case and Thompson, 1995).

This approach to identifying competence does, however, have strong face validity, appearing to take account of complexity and variability and including the person and situation in the process of measuring competence.

Competence and subconscious knowledge

The cognitive tradition is discussed in the writings of philosophers such as Polanyi, who explores concepts of knowledge and understanding. His work addresses the concepts of tacit knowledge – the human ability to recognize, understand and respond to features of a situation without being aware of this ability (Polanyi, 1958, 1967). Polanyi believes that all human knowledge has a tacit dimension which it is not possible to bring to the level of conscious functioning, but which nevertheless underpins much of an individual's conscious action and thought. Embedded in his theory is a concept of intuitive knowledge: the ability to know, without being aware of the knowledge and to act because of this deep-seated knowledge.

Schön (1991, 1993) applies Polanyi's ideas to developing professional competence. In particular, Schön asserts that competent professional practitioners 'exhibit a kind of knowing-in-practice which is tacit' (1991: viii) and demonstrate an ability to reflect on intuitive knowledge during their practical actions. Schön contends that an instrumental 'technical-rationalist' means–end approach is unable to encompass the initial need for framing problems experienced by many professionals. It is, therefore, he argues, inadequate as an approach for identifying competence. He proposes a model of professional practice which incorporates what he calls 'professional artistry' (1991: 268) and reflection in action (online decision making) during professional work. Professional artistry includes the largely tacit framing of situations in order to create a definable (even if ill-defined) problem to be addressed. His model encompasses unconscious and conscious aspects of behaviour.

There are a number of critiques of Schön's work, of which the most complete is that by Eraut (1994). Eraut suggests that Schön's theory has a number of defensible elements. He agrees that ill-defined situations require creative thinking, professionals draw on practical experience in an intuitive manner at the same time as reflecting on their actions, and reflection in action is embedded in this process. Eraut is less convinced by many of the cases used by Schön to exemplify his theory and suggests that Schön's work is best seen as contributing to theory of meta-cognition in professional practice.

Competence on a continuum

Some models of professional competence have their roots in the field of artificial intelligence and the development of expert systems which can mirror human thinking and decision making. One influential example of this is the work of Dreyfus and Dreyfus (1986). They present the concept of competence as a point on a continuum of professional development. They chart five steps in the progress from novice to expert, these being: novice, advanced beginner, competent, proficient and expert. The 'novice' can recognize features of a task, so that he or she can follow the rules, but is unable to go beyond them. This is typical of the student in the first or early second year of a speech and language therapy course, who rigidly applies a formula but does not know what to do if something goes wrong. The 'novice' has no coherent overall sense of a task. The 'advanced beginner' uses experience as well as rules to allow slight variations in a task: the student still does not have an overview of what they are looking for or trying to do and still sticks to the 'rules', but interprets them a little. At the level of 'competence', there is a reducing reliance on rules, and more reliance on integrating knowledge and skills. There is the ability to analyse a situation, organize approaches to a problem and vary behaviour in order to achieve not just one task, but overall success (e.g. in client management). What is still missing is a sense of what is important.

Dreyfus and Dreyfus consider competence to be the climax of rule-guided learning, where behaviour has not yet become the semi-automatic reflexive behaviour of the proficient practitioner. Beyond competence come levels of 'proficiency' and 'expertise', by which time the entire process is internalized with a development towards so-called 'intuitive' decision making.

Competence in speech and language therapy

Speech and language therapy, in common with many other professions, has produced a number of publications considering aspects of professional competence, and despite the fact that they are not always referred to explicitly, the theoretical approaches outlined above have had some influence on these publications.

Gailey (1988) presented a discussion on the nature and development of clinical competence and expertise. RCSLT issued its first professional standards guidelines in 1991. Stengelhofen (1984, 1993) investigated therapists' use of their theoretical bases in practice. van der Gaag and Davies (1992a,b) and Kamhi (1995) published papers on the knowledge, skills and attitudes of speech and language therapists. Roulstone (1995, 2001) presents a multi-modal approach to identifying speech and language therapy expertise in diagnosis and evaluation of children's communication disorders, and Williamson is developing a 'competencies framework' funded by RCSLT (Williamson, 2000, 2001, 2002).

Gailey suggested that there was a working consensus on the nature of professional competence in the speech and language therapy profession which was only just at the point (1988) where this was being formalized. The work of the professional body which she described resulted in the first comprehensive professional standards guidelines for speech and language therapists in the UK: *Communicating Quality* (CQ) (CSLT, 1991; RCSLT, 1996a). While not addressing what 'competence' is explicitly, CQ provides a code of ethics and guidance on client groups, the working context, the responsibilities of the speech and language therapist, and the service provider.

Stengelhofen (1984, 1993) developed a model of professional practice (see Figure 1.1) where each level influenced the others and all were influenced by the professionals' experience.

The model incorporates details of each of these levels, which could be used as a basis for measuring surface output (performance) and knowledge and attitude bases (competence, in her terms), although, as presented, the model was still at a high level of abstraction. Drawing on Schön's work, Stengelhofen hypothesized that clinicians utilized much of their theoretical knowledge tacitly, without drawing it to the forefront of their cognitive and linguistic rationalizing in clinical practice.

van der Gaag and Davies' work on competence (1992a,b; Davies and van der Gaag 1992a,b) addressed the question of:

> whether the knowledge and skills base of existing professionals was necessary and sufficient for the demands of contemporary health services. (Davies and van der Gaag, 1992a: 210)

This work complements that of Stengelhofen, in that, while hers involved direct observation and in-depth interviews with small numbers, van der Gaag and Davies included a total of almost 700 speech and language

Surface level	TECHNIQUES AND PROCEDURES: Includes skills in interpersonal relationships	
First deep level	KNOWLEDGE AND UNDERSTANDING: Speech and language pathology Linguistic knowledge Psychological knowledge Child development knowledge Sociological knowledge Clinical medicine knowledge KNOWLEDGE AWARENESS	ALL LEVELS INFLUENCED BY: Life experience Undergraduate learning Work experience Continuing education Relationship with employing authority
Second deep level (giving meaning to what is done and influencing use of knowledge and techniques and procedures)	ATTITUDES TO: Relationships with clients Relationships with parents Relationships with other professionals Relationships with employer Planning and evaluation Professional work and career future	Working context (e.g. school, clinic, etc.)
	MORAL VALUES	

Figure 1.1 Stengelhofen's model of professional practice.

therapists at some point in their consultation process. van der Gaag and Davies found a strong consensus about speech and language therapy knowledge and skills base at a super-ordinate level, with additional domain-specific knowledge requirements dependent on the contexts in which therapists work (Table 1.2). They also noted that some skills called for a complex integration of knowledge and practical application, concluding that speech and language therapists needed to draw on their knowledge base in order to work effectively with clients.

Table 1.2 Super-ordinate domains of knowledge and skill required by a competent speech and language therapist.

Knowledge	Speech and language Psychology Medicine Education policy Client and service management
Skill	Therapeutic Teaching Psychological Client and service management

van der Gaag and Davies also investigated the attitude base considered to be essential to competent practice in speech and language therapy. They noted that attitudes are considerably more difficult to measure than clinical skills, but they found a strong consensus on the core (Table 1.3), although they were not able to separate out attitudes and attributes.

Table 1.3 Core attitude base required by a competent speech and language therapist.

Desire to learn
Flexibility
Empathy
Positiveness
Professionalism
Self-awareness
Enthusiasm

van der Gaag and Davies' work is supported by that of Kamhi (1995) from the US. He identified four areas of 'clinical expertise' drawn from samples of clinicians and students working in a variety of clinical settings. Of these areas, knowledge, technical skills and interpersonal skills/attitudes match those identified by Stengelhofen, and van der Gaag and Davies very closely, while 'clinical philosophies' indicated an underlying values base which would support practice.

Roulstone's (1995, 2001) work took concepts of developing speech and language therapy competence and expertise a stage further. She describes a study on clinical decision making in which she aimed to find the answers to a number of questions about how practising speech and language therapists worked. First, she used the Dreyfus brothers' model (Dreyfus and Dreyfus, 1986) to consider the clinicians' levels of expertise. Next, she discussed the structure of clinical tasks in terms of complexity and ambiguity. She then identified aspects of the social and institutional context in which a clinician works, such as the level of detail available in referral information, availability of equipment and the amount of time available for client contacts. Depending on the relative stability of the clinician's work she then applied Schön's (1991) concepts of reflective practice. Finally, she noted the influence of clinicians' personal ideologies: their attitudes to their work.

The outcome of the study was an algorithm for clinical reasoning in work with paediatric cases, which could be used by students or clinicians. A child's presenting communication difficulties and clinical history are balanced against his or her current context in order to decide the level of priority to assign to the case. Roulstone stresses that the decision-making process in clinical work is necessarily at a high level of complexity which resists being broken down into easily identifiable chunks of skill.

The UK speech and language therapy professional body, RCSLT, is currently funding a project designed to establish the 'competencies' needed to practise as a speech and language therapist (Williamson, 2000, 2001).

The project has involved a wide range of consultation across the UK. Williamson identifies super-ordinate categories of speech and language therapy work (clinical work, research, training, management, supervision, mentoring) and contextualizes these in terms of 'core competencies' (needed by all speech and language therapists) and 'specific and differentiating competencies' needed in differing working roles and contexts.

Williamson's (2001) model appears to match closely the Australian approach to competence, with 'current competence' directly related to the speech and language therapist's existing post, but embedded within a broader area of 'capacity' (see Figure 1.2). In addition, 'competencies' are identified at the levels of task, process and judgement, and decision making (Figure 1.3), with the judgement and decision-making competencies being identified as being the least visible, but most important and hardest to measure.

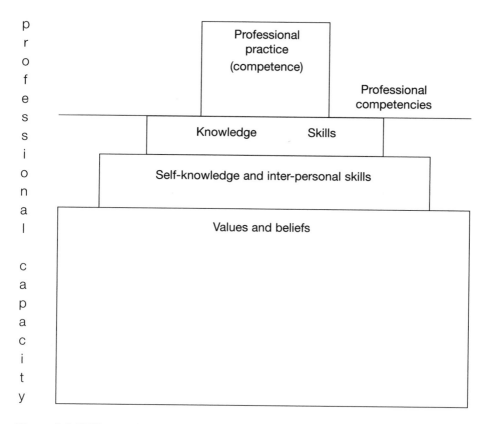

Figure 1.2 Williamson's competency framework model.

These speech and language therapy publications on competence have the common aim of attempting to make explicit the nature of competence in the profession. The studies described all make an attempt to identify the nature of competence and all identify similar super-ordinate structures of

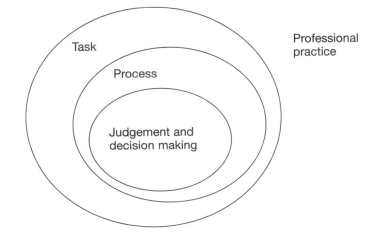

Figure 1.3 Cross-section of Williamson's professional practice level.

knowledge, skill and attitude as the component parts of competence. All the authors found skill (and especially technical skill) the easiest aspect of competence to identify, but also the least characteristic aspect of competence in itself. All of them considered a person's attitude and/or attributes to be a key to competent clinical practice. And all of the authors were in agreement that competence is easier to recognize than it is to describe, and this is a challenge for speech and language therapy education.

Competence and speech and language therapy education

Speech and language therapy is a graduate entry profession with courses offered by 15 universities in the UK. Bines (1992) presents a set of three models of professional education: pre-technocratic; technocratic; and post-technocratic (Table 1.4).

A pre-technocratic model is largely equated with apprenticeship. The technocratic model is one where learning is incorporated within universities, with three strands to student learning:

- acquisition of a knowledge base
- in-house application of this knowledge to practical issues within the HEI
- supervised practice on placements.

The third, post-technocratic, model emphasizes the development of competences through experience of, and reflection on, practice, with the placement being the central point of learning.

Stengelhofen (1984) suggested that speech and language therapy education in the mid-1980s fitted directly into Bines' (1992) 'technocratic'

Table 1.4 Bines' models of professional education.

Model	Characteristics
Pre-technocratic	Practical routines Mastery of facts and routines Workplace learning. Experienced practitioners act as instructors Employer-dominated learning/ national curriculum
Technocratic	Systematic knowledge base Academic subject specialists plus former practitioners deliver HEI-based curriculum Interpretation of knowledge base and development of 'principles and practice' Supervised workplace practice Experienced practitioners act as practice supervisors; HEI controls academic course content Tension between academic rigour and professional relevance
Post-technocratic	Knowledge for practice Acquisition of professional competences Systematic reflection on practice Practical dominates the curriculum Professional practitioner-educators operate in HEI and practice setting Subject specialists have negotiated role based on professional credibility or research Partnership between HEI and employers through learning contracts

Source: Bines (1992: 14–15).

model, while her aspiration was a reduction of the reliance on a discipline-based curriculum and a move towards a process-orientated curriculum in line with Bines' post-technocratic model. Over ten years later, Eastwood (1995) concluded that speech and language therapy courses still largely failed to present a coherent process-based approach to the 'theory of therapy', or developing clinical competence (although her analysis of the interview data she presents can be disputed). She, like Stengelhofen, recommended changes to the curriculum, moving away from a fact-based curriculum towards a learning-based one, again firmly embedded in Bines' (1992) post-technocratic model of professional education.

Speech and language therapy curriculum content as such has retained the same broad discipline areas since formal accreditation of courses was established (Segre, 1950; RCSLT, 2000). Current course documentation held at RCSLT does, however, demonstrate a significant difference from that reported by Stengelhofen and Eastwood. The focus and balance of course content has changed considerably since (and probably at least in part as a result of) the work of those authors. In many courses, the role of disciplines has been substantially reduced and the focus of the curriculum is increasingly applied to the process of speech and language therapy, specifically in order to achieve the development of academic and professional competence acknowledged in all stated course aims (Stansfield, 2001). Speech and language therapy education appears, at least as shown in course documentation, to be approaching Bines' post-technocratic model.

Education, competence, and the views of speech and language therapists

How do today's speech and language therapists identify competence in the pre-qualifying student? In order to compare 'real-life' experiences with the literature on competence and professional education, the following sections descibe a study by Stansfield (2001) of the views of three groups of speech and language therapy 'stakeholders'.

Clinicians, especially those close to educational establishments, are often involved in course design and in the clinical education of the next generation of their profession. Academics are involved in the design and delivery of degree courses and may supervise students on placement, but they rely on external clinical placements to deliver a major element of student learning. Students have an immediate personal interest in the range and quality of their courses as these influence not only their degree qualification, but also their future professional lives.

In Stansfield's study, semi-structured interviews were used to ask three groups of respondents with an interest in the field of student education to reflect on that aspect of their work. Respondents were 12 clinicians supervising students on placement, 12 academics lecturing on university courses and 14 students. These respondents were drawn from regions across England and Scotland and altogether had knowledge of 13 of the 15 universities offering speech and language therapy degrees. Respondents were interviewed in their own work or study bases, either individually or in groups of two or three. All interviews were audiotape-recorded and each interview took between one and one and a half hours. Following the interview, each tape was transcribed and typed. Respondents were sent their own transcripts for amendment, approval and permission to use the data. Once the transcripts were returned, data from the interviews were analysed using Glaser's (1992) approach to grounded theory. Each respondent was assigned a code of group-identifier letters and two randomly derived digits (e.g. ST11, student; CL26, clinician; AC03, academic) so that anonymity could be assured. The resulting themes are reported below.

Competence and clinical knowledge

Theory for practice

Clinical knowledge was a core concept of clinical competence for respondents, who all described broad, holistic and integrative concepts of knowledge. Theory from all the discipline areas identified by RCSLT (2000) was identified as continuing to be essential for the education of speech and language therapists. There was also a strong consensus that discipline knowledge changes, and as theory moves forward there is a need for the clinician to continue to learn and apply new theories. Possibly as a result, there was a large amount of reference to models (for example the PALPA model (Kay et al., 1992) and the Bloom and Lahey model (Lahey, 1988)), to provide educational frameworks for developing clinical knowledge and understanding of particular communication disorders. In addition, academics explicitly mentioned models of learning drawn from the educational literature and described how teaching was structured to enable students to understand their personal approaches to learning as well as to ground the theoretical aspects of their course.

Students made strong pleas for the relevance of discipline-based knowledge to clinical work to be made explicit. They could see the point of studying aspects of their course (all respondents saw discipline knowledge as necessary), but it was often only when it was applied in the clinical situation that its relevance, and therefore educational value as a part of competence, was acknowledged.

Theory in practice

Beyond the existence of discipline knowledge, there was a recognition that students need to use this knowledge in practice, giving rise to another form of 'knowing'. Theory and practice were seen by all respondents as key, interacting elements of competence, with practice enabling theory to come to life for students, and also allowing them to generate their own theories about practice. Clinicians initially appeared to see 'theory' as research- or discipline-based. They were, however, discriminating in their evaluation of theory, and in exploring the theories used in clinical work many of the clinicians identified ways in which they developed their own approaches, even if they were cautious about referring to these as theories.

> In therapy you have people talking about convoluted theories, but when you ask them what they would do, they say just what you would do yourself. It's linking theory that is important in working out what is going on with a child. (CL94)

Clinical theorizing (for example establishing hypotheses, testing these and involving the client in the decision-making process) was described explicitly by academic respondents, possibly because of their need to relate their clinical thinking to formal lecturing. In addition, the development of theory from practice was mentioned by a number of students as a part of their clinical placements:

> After my last placement I think I have got a theory of my own therapy. Until I was asked why I had done things I was really unaware of it. ... The therapist asked me what I got from that [session] – and she drew up this big chart of things – and I thought, 'wow, I observed all that!' I'd been far more organized about it than I thought I was. (ST97)

Students and academic respondents appeared most comfortable with the vocabulary of hypothesis testing, but in their different ways, the clinicians also demonstrated a firmly grounded understanding of how they developed their personal theories of practice. Unlike Eastwood's (1995) claims, respondents had a clear view of how their personal knowledge base included a knowledge of the process of therapy and individual constructs of clinical work, built on their personal interpretations of both discipline and process knowledge. Education to develop clinical knowledge was, therefore, seen as a complex construct, comprising theory for practice and theory in practice.

Clinical skill

Technical skill

There was a high level of consensus on the basic skills required to practise as a speech and language therapist, although without context, many skills (see Table 1.5) could be said to apply to almost any occupation involving work with people.

Table 1.5 Skills necessary for competent practice in speech and language therapy.

Ability to	collect data
	analyse data
	problem solve
	seek information
	use knowledge
	relate to people (especially clients) appropriately
	assess client's overall needs
	prepare for sessions
	use that preparation during sessions
	judge accurately how to proceed
	make onward referrals
	write well
	be flexible
	think on one's feet
	cope with new situations
	incorporate new learning
	do clinical research

Narrative from one student helped to identify the role of technical skills on a placement:

> I was able to run the Reynell comprehension section, just after we had had lectures on how to do it. You tend to remember things like 'non-contingent praise'. I found it really useful. I was petrified when I started doing it, as I was warned the child wouldn't cooperate. It was a big relief when he actually did it. I thought 'Oh, I can do this; put the equipment out; I can record the answers; I can score it'. It really built up my confidence. ... To a certain extent it was intuitive, ... talking to children anyway, but we had actually had the lectures on the type of praise to use and the way to encourage children, so it was making sure that everything I said was along the same lines. I think I had the technical skills to do the test. (ST11)

Some students had a view of skilled clinical action as a challenging goal. ST71 stated that 'on a personal level, you need to have personal skills up to scratch', implying an absolute measurable level of interpersonal skill, while ST11 was clear that 'flexibility is important, but also competence is about being right'.

'Competencies' were mentioned by many of the respondents in relation to clinical skills. Course or clinic literature which had been prepared to identify 'competencies' in students was found to be a helpful way of identifying the necessary skills for students and clinicians at given points in a course. Techniques and measurable competencies were on the whole, however, seen as being necessary, but not sufficient for skilled practice. Clinical skills were seen by all respondents as being more complex than a straightforward list of 'can do' technical activities and the list (Table 1.5) generated in the course of the interviews was heavily contextualized. Several respondents echoed AC03 when she said, in discussing skilled clinical action, that it 'is more than just the sum of the parts. It is not just a list of the parts'. Thus an NVQ approach to identifying competence in the speech and language therapy student is not seen as being the way forward.

Flexibility

While all the skill areas listed in Table 1.5 were considered to be necessary for competent clinical performance, an essential component mentioned by every respondent was flexibility. It was identified as underpinning every successful session and its absence was usually seen to be a part, if not all, of the cause of unsuccessful ones. One student reported finding it especially difficult to be flexible enough to make rapid decisions during a session. 'It is difficult to think "on the hoof". I think this will speed up with practice. It is a result of lack of practice and confidence' (ST72). As part of their clinical education, most students described being taught techniques to build flexibility into their sessions before this became embedded in their practice. ST45, for example, said 'As part of our placement preparation, in our session plan we are encouraged to plan an easier and a harder task for each goal in case we need to adjust an activity.' Other students described situations where they had needed to be flexible, together with the reasons why this was more or less easy, for example:

> It is hard not to be rigid. I had a session where a client broke down in tears. At first I though 'oh no, I've got all this work to get through'. It was a single-session evaluation [degree practical assessment] and it was important to me, because there was a viva afterwards. Then I just thought – no, I was there for that person so I needed to step back and look at what was going on and be in tune with that time, and adapt to suit them and forget your plan. What is important for that person at that time might not be their word-finding or whatever. This lady was telling me about what had happened to her in the past. We went with that and then discussed what she wanted to do after she had disclosed her feelings. That was what she needed. (ST48)

In this session, flexibility was essential because of the behaviour of the client, even though the situation and the student's limited experience made flexibility difficult.

Clinical skill and knowledge

When discussing skilled clinical work, clinicians and academics tended to describe principles of intervention, rather than actual events. They obviously possessed deep-seated clinical knowledge when they described how they planned and then changed their own sessions, but such decision making may be difficult to explain to students. Narrative from one clinician gives an example of this:

> In the waiting room I am looking at what they [child] look like: physical skills; how they are interacting with mum; what they are like when they come through to the [therapy] room. These give a really good starting point for the rest of my session. It varies from child to child and depending on the mum.
>
> The more experience I have had, the quicker I make decisions.
>
> I have a checklist in my head in order of sections I want to look at – pre-linguistics or language, depending on the age of the child. I want an answer in my head before I let them go at the end of the session. (CL26)

At first clinicians and academics variously described their decisions on how to conduct sessions as on-the-spot decision making, gut instinct or intuition. Once respondents reflected on this, however, intuition was *not* seen to be a major part of skilled clinical decision making. The majority of qualified speech and language therapists, while acknowledging that online decision making was difficult to articulate, identified the importance of having learned from previous mistakes and an increasing ability to notice things and integrate them into their existing knowledge base as core aspects of competent practice. They also recognized the need to help students to achieve the same abilities to combine skill and knowledge.

It was clear from respondents that knowledge and skill were not seen in isolation. Templates of previous clients (depending on the length of experience of the clinician) were complemented by such things as local sociological knowledge (for example the typical performance on standardized assessments in given areas of a city) and theoretical underpinnings (e.g. ages and stages of development; theories of approach to different communication disorders), thus fitting the models described by Dreyfus and Dreyfus (1986) and Roulstone (2001). In acknowledging the difficulties of enabling students to achieve this level of decision making most respondents agreed with CL26 when she said:

> You start thinking it is all intuition but forget there is a theory behind it all and you have forgotten what you have learned and where you are coming from. (CL26)

Confidence and clinical skill

Lack of confidence and fear were all mentioned by students as a part of their clinical experience. On the whole, fear was exemplified by descriptions of one-off events, but it was a strong theme and appeared to interfere with students' ability to use their knowledge and be flexible in their clinical interactions:

> It is terrifying going out and doing it. It's worse when someone is breathing down your neck and watching everything you do. (ST91)

Academics and clinicians were all aware of the fear aspect of clinic for students. For example, 'Students perceive all new cases as a "physical jolt" but that is fear!' (AC7). Structured learning was seen to be a major contributing factor in reducing fear. Academic staff provided an overview of placement organization, indicating how the placement experience was planned across speech and language therapy courses and integrated with the university-based learning to facilitate development of confidence and competence. Clinicians were also keen to demonstrate how they organized placement experience for the benefit of students. For example:

> There is a 'pathway' used by all our clinicians who work with students. It involves learning contracts, information about their past experience of placements. We set up observation records, which the therapist carries out at least three times with each student. Students set out their learning goals with learning contracts. (CL96)

All students valued support from therapists in developing their confidence and it was not exclusively the 'gentle' approach that was identified as being helpful.

> I like clinicians who tell the truth rather than patronising – overloading with praise for one small thing you have done right. You know there is a process of first positive, then criticism of negative points. I like to be treated not totally like a student, but as a fellow professional so you can exchange information. (ST17)

> A clinician needs to be more than nice and supportive. (ST49)

Clinicians also recognized the need for constructive criticism, although they also acknowledged the difficulties in this.

> It is easy for a student to become really hurt and devastated by something which is not really such a big issue. Things can get out of proportion. It is hard giving them structured help and not destroying them. (CL35)

All groups of respondents identified one element of the supervisory process which created tensions: that is, the need for clinicians to act not only as facilitators of students' learning and confidence, but also as assessors of competence. Clinicians welcomed students who suggested their own ideas: 'If they want to disagree [with me] I think that is great, so long as they can justify what they say' (CL44). But students were acutely aware of this dichotomy of roles and the consequent caution needed in their willingness to accept or challenge clinicians' judgements.

Nevertheless, students' clinical skill was seen to be facilitated by confidence, and this is developed especially when a student and clinician are able to 'get along' on a personal level. The relationship between student and clinician was identified as being important in developing confidence. Academics, clinicians and students all identified inter-personal relationships as a foundation upon which other aspects of clinical learning and the development of confidence and competence could build.

Personal characteristics

Respondents were clear that in order to be competent, a speech and language therapist has to be a 'people person' and that the profession appears to attract individuals with a basic interest in people. An initial list of personal characteristics considered necessary for competent practice was generated relatively easily (see Table 1.6). The majority of characteristics deemed to be desirable were 'gentle' (van der Gaag and Davies, 1992b), people-based attitudes, values and attributes, although it was acknowledged that there may be a change in the characteristics which could be desirable as the work of the profession changed.

As with the skills listed earlier, the majority of these 'desirable' characteristics exist in much work involving people. All were mentioned by a number of respondents, with the key characteristics identified by the majority being enthusiasm and motivation. From these, other characteristics appeared to follow. One student spoke of a clinician who 'was really motivated herself. She really loved her work. I would like to be like her'

Table 1.6 Personal characteristics and competence.

Desirable		Undesirable
Good communicator	Enthusiastic	Poor communicator
Pleasant	Motivated	Uncaring
Warm	Positive	Disinterested
Supportive	Flexible	Cynical
Able to instil confidence	Curious	Patronising
Empathetic	(interested in	Aloof
Able to read situations	learning)	Unapproachable
accurately	Insightful	Critical without offering
Genuinely interested in	Having a good	support
the clients/students	self-knowledge	Lacking confidence
Sensitive to clients'	Conscientious	Disorganized
needs	Having integrity	Lazy
Accepting of clients'	Reliable	
views	Honest	
Considerate	Patient	
Encouraging	Professional	

(ST48). Another, while listing many positive aspects of a clinician, said 'and especially she was enthusiastic' (ST72). Clinicians and academics, similarly, spoke of good students as being, for example, 'interested, aware, motivated' (CL35).

The identification of desirable and undesirable personal characteristics listed in Table 1.6 was the beginning, but not the end of the story, as could be seen when respondents were asked to describe their most memorable clinician or student. About half of the memorable individuals were highly commended, while the other half were criticized in strong terms. All the descriptions focused predominantly on the attitudes and attributes of the person in question, rather than what they knew or could do. It was not, however, only the presence or absence of these characteristics but also their amount and intensity. The qualifying vocabulary used by respondents demonstrated the strength of feeling underlying these responses.

Students spoke of positive experience of clinicians with 'a genuine interest in the person. ... A very good listener. ... An excellent role model' (ST14); 'the one who stands out was really motivated herself' (ST48); 'she gave brilliant feedback ...' (ST97). Negative experience was also emphatically described: '*so* disorganized' (ST17); 'rude and unprofessional' (ST47); 'aloof, unapproachable' (ST71). Clinicians similarly saw intensity as being an issue. Memorable students were 'very interested ... they bring a joy and enthusiasm' (CL29); 'very lively ... bright and bubbly ... would be good at whatever she did' (CL44). Negative experience was also a matter of degree:

> Partly it was personality, but also the amount she asked of the clinician and the *way* she asked – demanding support. She was *constantly* there asking questions ... but she completely ignored the answers she was given. (CL26)

... no insight and very little initiative or interest shown ... wouldn't or couldn't ask questions. She seemed to have no motivation. ... Always came back with an excuse. (CL43)

Other respondents spoke of consideration which bordered on obsequiousness, enthusiasm and motivation which became intrusive over time, and an interest in learning which led to unsustainable demands on the clinical supervisor. In developing competence, therefore, it is clear that students have a fine line to tread. They are expected to be enthusiastic but not to excess, proactive but not pushy, assertive but not aggressive, knowledgeable but not a know-all, and confident and flexible (but not overconfident or over-flexible). It is easy to see that learning to judge the nuances of clinical behaviour is a challenging task and one which does not easily lend itself to clear guidelines or measurement. A person's overall stance is difficult to identify in behavioural terms, while still being highly influential, and many aspects of competence (for example being easy to talk to) are easier to recognize than to measure.

Learnability

It was clear from discussion with the respondents that enthusiasm and motivation develop alongside academic and practical knowledge and are reinforced by the level of confidence in this knowledge. These attitudes are also variable, according to whether the speech and language therapy student has confidence in his or her own abilities, the relationship with the clinician and whether he or she enjoys working with a particular client group, or in a particular clinical setting. As an example, a student may be highly motivated in work with autistic clients, but afraid of working with adults who stutter, or vice versa. In addition, it is the rare individual who is unfailingly enthusiastic, motivated and confident. Arguably, those who are may be demonstrating a lack of perception of situations, at least some of the time.

Some respondents described clinicians and students whose overall manner was seen as positive. Enthusiasm and empathy, for example, were seen as being not purely related to specific contexts, but 'of the person' in a broader sense. Thus, there did appear to be a view that a student's overall approach to life would colour his or her approach to work and influence his or her ability to become a competent clinician.

Student confidence can, however, be increased or decreased through subtle inter-personal interactions between student, client and/or clinician. These can give rise to emotional reactions which are often difficult for students to recognize in or admit to themselves, still less to others (clinicians or tutors). The emotional impact of positive and negative experiences of clinical placements can, however, have a significant effect on the student speech and language therapist's developing confidence and competence.

When asked if a therapist was 'born or made', there was a range of views on whether personal characteristics were innate attributes, as suggested by Spencer and Spencer (1993), or attitudes and values which could be learned and developed. Initially, the majority of respondents suggested that some personal characteristics were innate character traits but they were vague on which these might be. Once this concept of aptitude for the work was teased out a little, respondents agreed that most, if not all, of the attitude and value base of the profession could be learned by students, given an appropriate level of support and an appropriate personal attitude to learning. Learnability was seen to depend on students' experiences across their course and clinicians' approaches to the learning environment in clinic. Learning to acquire the attitudes and values of competent speech and language therapy practice was thus recognized as being far less tangible than learning how to acquire knowledge and skill, while being closely related to these aspects of competence.

Modelling the development of competence in speech and language therapy education

Respondents' views on developing clinical competence in the speech and language therapy student appeared at first to fall into the relatively traditional subcategories of knowledge, skills and personal characteristics (attributes, values and attitudes) identified by previous authors. On further analysis, these simple categories were found to have considerable depth of meaning for respondents. Competent clinical practice is seen as being complex and determined by context. It is the result of an interaction between discipline and process knowledge, practical and technical skills, and a personal stance which values clients and professional learning. It depends on the situation, the individuals present and the degree of confidence felt by the various participants in the clinical situation. As a result, there can be seen to be several layers within these concepts as shown in Model 1 (see Figure 1.4).

Throughout the interviews with respondents there emerged a consensus that students could become competent clinicians, given a basic level of motivation towards working with clients and towards learning. Weaknesses in some areas could usually be overcome by strengths in others and Model 1 suggests that the three super-ordinate aspects of competence – knowledge, skills and personal characteristics – are intimately related to each other and inter-dependent in the development of competence in students.

The identification of competence in speech and language therapy students is a complex process, made more complex by the fact that any discussion of competence is in danger of using a single vocabulary which means substantially different things to different people (e.g. Jessup, 1991; Spencer and Spencer, 1993; Eastwood, 1995; Williamson, 2002). Because

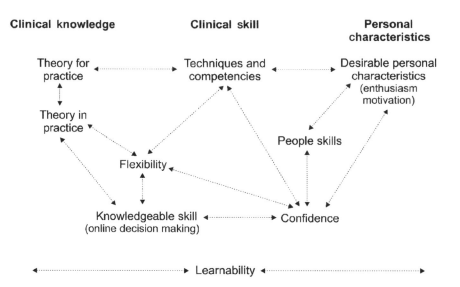

Figure 1.4 Model 1: development of competence in speech and language therapy.

there are so many dimensions to competence in speech and language therapy, and because it exists not in isolation, but in the context of the profession's continually changing working environment, there can be no static identification of what competence is. The literature on developing professional and clinical competence in speech and language therapy also demonstrates a dichotomy between the need to identify aspects of competence at particular points in a student's career, and a broader, more inclusive approach to competence, which involves continuing professional development. Communication between the various 'stakeholders' in speech and language therapy education is therefore an ongoing necessity. If students are to be educated successfully for practice, the various groups involved in that education need to communicate with each other on a regular and frequent basis, in order to explore each other's ideas, reach shared understandings and revisit older notions about the nature and development of competence.

Enhanced communication would have a number of benefits. First, it would allow each group to explore and increase their understanding of each other's priorities, the reasons for these priorities and the impact they have on speech and language therapists' perceptions of student competence. Second, it would allow a sharing of views on the nature of speech and language therapy professional competence itself and facilitate consensus on how this can be identified and measured (in terms of competencies (e.g. Williamson, 2001), if these are agreed). Third, it would allow speech and language therapists to explore and share their knowledge about the influences on the nature and development of competence. Fourth, as a result of these shared understandings, it would allow for decisions to be made on how best to facilitate the development of competence in pre-qualifying education. Flexibility, enthusiasm, motivation and confidence were identified by respondents as key aspects of competence in speech and language therapist work, but without context these qualities are meaningless. Shared communication between speech and language therapists can provide that professional context. It can help to identify the ways in which students can be educated to use their knowledge, skill and personal characteristics across a wide range of professional situations, increasing their ability to work professionally as a result.

Communication must be at several levels. It should be multidirectional, rather than involving simply one group or individual telling another what they consider to be needed. It should be ongoing, not simply formal training or a one-off event, and there needs to be continuity and re-initiation of communication on a regular and frequent basis if student learning is to receive priority.

The knowledge base will change, new approaches to therapy will require new skills and techniques, and the changing working environment may well demand changing personal characteristics in the speech and language therapy profession. Understandings will therefore also change, and consequently there is a need for ongoing, regular and frequent communication between academics, clinicians, students and others involved in clinical work to maintain shared understandings of the nature of competence in speech and language therapy, especially in the new graduate, and the ways in which this can be developed and measured throughout the course.

Conclusion

The literature reviewed and interviews with speech and language therapy respondents for this study highlighted the complexities inherent in describing competence. The vocabulary of competence and competencies was used frequently, but rarely defined. Respondents were, however, clear that competence in speech and language therapy is a holistic concept. It includes a defined, but rapidly changing knowledge base; a more broadly defined and rapidly changing skill base; an attitudes and values base which is apparently shared, but not explicit; and, possibly, predisposing innate personal attributes. Despite the difficulties in defining the exact nature of competence, it was agreed that it was possible to learn. Learning to become competent involves university-based and clinic-based education and support in order to achieve recognizable, competent, clinical practice.

Speech and language therapists need to be rounded human beings. Their education must allow them to develop their own critical faculties, applying knowledge, skills, their personal characteristics, personal experience and understanding to the field of speech and language therapy. As students, they will develop the intellectual capacity to engage with new ideas in a field where there are no easy or straightforward answers.

Speech and language therapy education must encompass linguistic, psychological, social and medical aspects of communication disability, at the same time as developing students' ability to act to reduce the impact of that disability for their clients. Speech and language therapy students learn individually defined skills, but these need to be incorporated rapidly into a broader competence base, raising difficulties for those who wish to quantify every aspect of a student's clinical learning and behaviour. Measurement of observable skills alone runs the risk of measuring only what can be easily quantified and disregarding the deeper cognitive structures involved in competent clinical performance. Model 1 gives some insight into the complexities involved in developing clinical competence. By the time a student graduates, many of the substructures of competence have been buried deep in the subconscious. They are no longer at the forefront of cognition and are not stored linguistically, but are embedded in the individual's tacit knowledge base.

The mark of the competent speech and language therapy graduate is the ability to use his or her capabilities in a wide range of contexts while responding to novel situations involving communication disability. Speech and language therapy education aims to enable the development of a graduate who achieves basic competence, but who also has the tools to continue to learn and change practice throughout his or her professional life.

References

Bines H (1992) Issues in course design. In Bines P, Watson D (eds) Developing Professional Education. Buckingham: Society for Research into Higher Education.

Case S, Thompson L (1995) Gender differences in student development: examining life stories, career histories and learning plans. In Boyatzis R, Cowen S, Kolb D et al. (eds) Innovation in Professional Education. San Francisco: Jossey-Bass.

College of Speech and Language Therapists (CSLT) (1991) Communicating Quality. London: CSLT.

Davies P, van der Gaag A (1992a) The professional competence of speech therapists I: introduction and methodology. Clinical Rehabilitation 6: 209–214.

Davies P, van der Gaag A (1992b) The professional competence of speech therapists III: skills and skill mix possibilities. Clinical Rehabilitation 6: 311–323.

Dreyfus HL, Dreyfus SE (1986) Mind Over Machine: The Power of Human Intuition and Expertise in the Era of the Computer. New York: The Free Press.

Eastwood J (1995) Therapy in the curriculum: Investigating an aspect of speech and language therapy education. Unpublished MPhil thesis, De Montfort University, Leicester.

Eraut M (1994) Developing Professional Knowledge and Competence. London: Falmer Press.

Gailey L (1988) Competence in speech therapy. In Ellis R (ed.) Professional Competence and Quality Assurance in the Caring Professions. London: Croom Helm.

Glaser B (1992) Emergence versus Forcing: Basics of Grounded Theory Analysis. Mill Valley, CA: Sociology Press.

Gonczi A (1994) Competency based assessment in the professions in Australia. Assessment in Education 1: 27–44.

Gonczi A, Hager P, Oliver L (1990) Establishing Competency-based Standards in the Professions. Canberra: Commonwealth of Australia.

Hager P, Hyland T (2002) Vocational education and training. In Blake N, Smeyers P, Smith R, Standish P (eds) The Blackwell Guide to the Philosophy of Education. London: Blackwell.

Jessup G (1991) Outcomes: NVQs and the Emerging Model of Education and Training. London: Falmer Press.

Kamhi A (1995) Research to practice. Defining, developing and maintaining clinical expertise. Language, Speech and Hearing Services in Schools 26: 353–356.

Kay J, Lesser R, Colthart M (1992) PALPA: Psycholinguistic Assessment of Language Processing in Aphasia. Hove: Lawrence Erlbaum Associates.

Lahey M (1988) Language Disorders and Language Development. London: Collier Macmillan.

Polanyi M (1958) Personal Knowledge. London: Routledge and Kegan Paul.

Polanyi M (1967) The Tacit Dimension. London: Routledge and Kegan Paul.

Roulstone S (1995) The child, the process, the expertise. Identification of priority children from pre-school referrals to speech and language therapy. Unpublished PhD thesis, Brunel University, London.

Roulstone S (2001) Consensus and variability between speech and language therapists in the assessment and selection of pre-school children for intervention: a body of knowledge or ideosyncratic decisions? International Journal of Language and Communication Disorders 36: 329–348.

Royal College of Speech and Language Therapists (RCSLT) (1996) Communicating Quality 2. London: RCSLT

Royal College of Speech and Language Therapists (RCSLT) (2000) Guidelines on the Accreditation of Courses Leading to a Qualification in Speech and Language Therapy. London: RCSLT.

Schön D (1991) The Reflective Practitioner: How Professionals Think in Action. Aldershot: Avebury Ashgate Publishers.

Schön D (1993) Educating the Reflective Practitioner. San Francisco: Jossey-Bass.

Segre R (1950) Present situation in logopaedics and phoniatrics in various countries. Folic Phoniatrica 2: 173–202.

Spencer LM, Spencer SM (eds) (1993) Competence at Work. Models for Superior Performance. New York: John Wiley.

Stansfield J (2001) Education for practice: the development of competence in speech and language therapy students. Unpublished EdD thesis, University of Durham.

Stengelhofen J (1984) Curricula for professional education: an investigation into theory and practice in the work of speech therapists. Unpublished MEd thesis, University of Birmingham.

Stengelhofen J (1993) Teaching Students in Clinical Settings. London: Chapman and Hall.

van der Gaag A, Davies P (1992a) The professional competence of speech therapists II: knowledge base. Clinical Rehabilitation 6: 215–224.

van der Gaag A, Davies P (1992b) The professional competence of speech therapists: IV: attitude and attribution base. Clinical Rehabilitation 6: 325–331.

Williamson K (2000) The best things for the best reasons. RCSLT Bulletin 582: 17–18.

Williamson K (2001) Capable, confident and competent. RCSLT Bulletin 592: 12–13.

Williamson K (2002) RCSLT competencies project. http//www.rcslt.org/com.shtml

Chapter 2
Case-based problem solving for speech and language therapy students

Anne Whitworth, Sue Franklin and Barbara Dodd

Introduction

The problem: the knowledge base of speech and language therapy is continually expanding and evolving as evidence develops, clinical populations diversify and contexts change. How do we create clinicians who will be able to respond actively to these changes throughout their career, providing effective services to their clients and continually developing their own skills? The traditional approach to the education of speech and language therapists does not encourage this kind of flexible learning ability. Like many academic programmes, the focus of education in this field has been one of acquiring knowledge via a predominantly lecture-based teaching strategy. However, the developments in reflective learning and problem-based learning (PBL) over the past two decades have shifted the focus of education to the learning process itself and aim to equip students with lifelong learning skills. In response to these developments in educational theory, core changes were made to the speech and language therapy curriculum at the University of Newcastle.

This chapter describes the development and implementation of a hybrid model of PBL for speech and language therapy students. Using a case-based problem-solving (CBPS) approach, core language pathology modules are taught using real-life cases, with students applying a systematic framework of problem solving to integrate theory and practice. A reorganization of the entire curriculum has facilitated integration of information from different disciplines in planning case management, and this is reinforced through a parallel framework used in clinical placements. While this approach has been introduced into both the four-year undergraduate and two-year postgraduate programmes, only its integration into the undergraduate programme will be outlined here. Measures are in place to assist in evaluating this programme.

A case-based problem-solving (CBPS) approach: the theoretical background

The philosophy underpinning the CBPS approach in Newcastle draws extensively on the literature and evidence emerging from PBL. While a debate exists as to whether a curriculum can successfully draw on principles and yet not adopt PBL in a pure form (Margetson, 1999; Maudsley, 1999), the Newcastle course developed from a need to balance the desirability of the educational philosophy with finite resources and as such is considered to be a hybrid of pure PBL.

Pure problem-based learning

'Problem-based learning is an approach to structuring the curriculum which involves confronting students with problems from practice which provide a stimulus for learning' (Boud and Feletti, 1991: 21). Through the process of solving real clinical problems, the problem-solving process itself provides an explicit framework from which to solve immediate and future problems, aiming to encourage self-directed learning where students are both motivated to learn and actively engaged in their own learning (see Boud and Feletti, 1991; Brandon and Majumdar, 1997, for overviews of PBL). The use of real problems is motivated by a belief that knowledge is best remembered in context. Real problems are also used to reactivate prior learned information so that this can be reorganized when integrating new information (Schmidt, 1993). Initially introduced into medical curricula in the mid-1970s (Neufeld and Barrows, 1974; Neufeld et al., 1989), PBL is now widely used throughout undergraduate medical education (Smits et al., 2002) and has been adopted within other health and non-health professional education. Health professions adopting PBL curricula include nursing (e.g. Biley and Smith, 1999), clinical psychology (e.g. Huey, 2001), occupational therapy (e.g. Sadlo, 1997), social work (e.g. Sable et al., 2001), dietetics (e.g. Dalton, 1999), dentistry (e.g. Fincham and Shuler, 2001), chiropractice (e.g. Bovee and Gran, 2000) and healthcare management (e.g. de Virgilio, 1993).

Courses adopting a pure PBL approach make exclusive use of a method whereby small groups of students take a problem provided by the course leader and seek to solve it through self-directed study and group discussion. All aspects of the curriculum are integrated to allow this to take place. The student groups meet under the supervision of a tutor, who enhances the process of learning but does not contribute expert or specialist knowledge. The degree to which courses have adopted pure PBL varies widely.

Does PBL work?

The effectiveness of PBL has been studied extensively with numerous studies reporting anecdotal and empirical evidence of a largely positive nature. Dolmans and Schmidt (1996) report the benefits of PBL as a greater retention of knowledge and information, enhanced integration of theory to practice, the fostering of greater interest in the subject matter of the course and the development of self-directed learning skills that equip students with a sound basis for lifelong learning and the application of new information. The learning approach allows for individuals' different learning needs and interests (Dolmans et al., 1993), and is also more enjoyable as a method of learning (Albanese and Mitchell, 1993; Dolmans and Schmidt, 1996; Bligh et al., 2000). Students, when asked to evaluate PBL in an occupational therapy curriculum, have reported benefits in managing information, critical reasoning, communication and team-building (Hammel et al., 1999).

Empirical evidence as to whether academic performance improves remains contentious. Verhoeven et al. (1998) compared the academic performance from two Dutch medical curricula, one offering a PBL programme and the other employing non-PBL methods. They found no overall systematic differences between the two groups. Ozuah et al. (2001) looked at the impact of PBL on medical residents' self-directed learning and found that, while the residents exposed to PBL engaged in significantly higher levels of self-directed learning than residents in a lecture-based course, the PBL group had returned to baseline levels of self-directed learning at the three-month follow-up, and any significant differences between the groups were no longer present. Colliver (2000) conducted a review of the literature and found no persuasive evidence that PBL improved either knowledge or clinical performance, and that effect sizes were small given the extensive resources required by a PBL curriculum. Similarly, Nandi et al. (2000) found that, while such areas as interpersonal skills, psychosocial knowledge and attitudes were all at a higher level following PBL, performance on science examinations was no different. Fincham and Shuler (2001), on the other hand, reported that dental students undertaking a pure PBL curriculum performed significantly better than peers exposed to a traditional lecture-based curriculum. These studies suggest that, while acquisition of the knowledge base may or may not be enhanced by the approach, there appear to be numerous other benefits for graduates from a PBL programme. The more positive learning environment has also been considered a worthy benefit of PBL for students and staff alike (Albanese, 2000). If, however, the importance of PBL is in helping clinicians develop through their working lives, then the proof of PBL's efficacy will be found in long-term follow-up. Many programmes are currently involved in collecting these data.

Hybrid models of PBL

Proponents of pure PBL argue that the term has been applied loosely with, for example, 'PBL courses' adopting PBL only within single subjects, confounding the evidence base and blurring the essential elements of good practice in PBL (Maudsley, 1999). Nevertheless, hybrid programmes have emerged and report varying degrees of success. Armstrong (1991) strongly defends the hybrid curriculum established in the Harvard Medical School as achieving its pedagogical objectives. Miller et al. (2000) similarly defend an alternatively structured yet reportedly successful model based around case studies and PBL principles, as do Dowd and Davidhizar (1999), who stress the advantage of using real-world problems while not adapting the curriculum extensively. Among the difficulties experienced with hybrid courses are reported instances of 'mini-lecturing', unsatisfactory group dynamics and student frustration with non-expert tutors (Houlden et al., 2001). Consequently, hybrid programmes need to be continually monitored to evaluate their effectiveness. The speech and language therapy programme in Newcastle considers ongoing evaluation as an essential component of the curriculum revision process. Our programme does, however, demonstrate that an adaptation of a pure approach can offer an alternative where resources do not permit a pure approach to be implemented.

The context for implementation: the course review

The intention to reform the learning approach used in our curriculum was in the context of a planned revision of the entire curriculum of the speech and language therapy programme at the University of Newcastle. This decision was driven by three major factors. Two were pragmatic. First, the conversion to a modular structure, required by the University, meant that credit values for subjects no longer matched content. Second, student (and staff) contact hours were excessive, additional subjects having been added over the years to cover new topics, wherever they fitted in the timetable. The course had consequently lost the cohesion and coherence of its original design. The third and primary reason, however, was the students' perception that theoretical knowledge and clinical practice were separate. Their clinical practice reflected what they had experienced on clinical placement, irrespective of their grasp of theory that they demonstrated in written assessment.

The aims of the new curriculum were not unlike those of many other speech and language therapy programmes. The graduates were to have:

- an in-depth understanding of current knowledge of the causes, symptomatology and consequences of the range of human communication disorders and the clinical skills necessary for cost-effective intervention practice
- research abilities that will allow them to build the knowledge base of a relatively recent discipline and to meet employers' need for graduates able to validly evaluate clinical service provision

- the conceptual tools to enable them to effectively adapt to advances in theory and developments in clinical practice throughout their working lives
- the necessary knowledge and skills to act as advocates for their profession and the population they will serve as speech and language therapists.

The following process was adopted for the curriculum review. A meeting of all departmental staff agreed the need to revise the curriculum. Relevant data were assembled, both from other courses in the UK and overseas, and from questionnaires completed by current and past students of the Newcastle course, local clinical supervisors and employers. A Course Review Consultative Committee (CRCC) was set up, comprising members of the department of speech academic staff, student representatives, managers of speech and language therapy services, a representative of the NHS Executive's Northern and Yorkshire Office and the dean of education. The role of the CRCC was to provide a framework for the new undergraduate and postgraduate clinical courses. Specifically, the CRCC determined: (a) a conceptual framework that would allow students to organize the information presented; (b) the general learning goals for each year of the courses; and (c) how the principles of PBL may be applied to the course.

The key changes arising from the CRCC's discussion were:

- *Use of a behavioural rather than a medical model for presenting information.* Subjects were reorganized around aspects of language/communication rather than diagnostic categories (with some exceptions, e.g. cleft palate, dysfluency). Acquired and developmental disorders were therefore integrated within, for example, core speech and language pathology modules, and many of these modules were then team-taught by specialists from both paediatric and adult fields.
- *Research skills taught throughout the course.* The ability to evaluate clinical efficacy for individual cases, audit service provision and read relevant research literature critically is encouraged by research skills subjects in all four years of the course.
- *Learning approaches that emphasized the link between theory and practice.* The CBPS approach was developed and introduced to all speech and language pathology modules, which then became the central focus of the course. Modules that did not adopt this approach included, for example, anatomy, physiology and phonetics.

The final draft of the new curriculum, after scrutiny by staff and the CRCC, was submitted to the University Teaching Committee and to The Royal College of Speech and Language Therapists Academic Board for approval. The first two years of the new curriculum were implemented in 1998 and the second two years in 1999. The first cohort of students educated entirely by the new curriculum graduated in 2002.

Overall CBPS course structure

The CBPS components of the course were structured as follows, with different years of the course corresponding to stages 1 to 4.

- **Stage 1**: the concept of PBL is introduced in clinical education at the beginning of the course. Two simple cases (one a phonetic articulation disorder and one of dysarthria) are introduced in the second semester.
- **Stage 2**: the links between theory and practice (including application of linguistic analysis skills) are made explicit by the CBPS teaching of developmental and acquired disorders of phonology, sentence processing and semantics throughout the second year.
- **Stage 3**: the pragmatic module adopts a similar framework to the second year modules, while specific diagnoses and disorders (dysfluency, voice, laryngectomy, cleft palate, cerebral palsy, hearing impairment, autism, intellectual impairment, dementia, head injury) are taught intensively, using a range of learning approaches that include both CBPS and lecture-based courses.
- **Stage 4**: the final year focuses on professional competence. This includes developing the ability to manage novel individual cases (with minimal supervision) and to participate in service provision in a wider context (service policy implementation, case conferences, clinic administration, quality assurance statistics). The course-work strand of stage 4 supports the acquisition of clinical competence by providing a course focusing on professional issues (e.g. medico-legal requirements, service provision policies of different providers in health and education) and by presenting students with CBPS exercises of complex, novel cases or caseloads. Table 2.1 sets out the broad goals for the academic and clinical learning throughout the four years.

Table 2.1 Overall goals for each year of the course.

Stage	Academic	Clinical
1	Foundation knowledge	Observers
2	Integrators	Analysts
3	Critical thinkers	Clinicians
4	Clinical scientists	Professionals

What is a CBPS approach?

There are two mechanisms in the approach. These involve, first, the decision process involved in solving a problem and, second, the case-based problem framework. What we tell the students is this:

Every case that you assess is unique. Consequently there are no recipes that can be generally applied to a particular diagnostic group or age of child. Further clinical management involves more than simply planning a course of therapy. Any case that is referred to a speech and language therapist for assessment poses a problem that needs to be solved. To solve that problem, the clinician needs to apply a systematic problem-solving approach.

Decision process

Students are exposed to a model of problem solving involving eight steps. These are loosely aligned with the pure PBL model.

- *Step 1: Explore and define the problem.* The problem is defined, involving clarification of all terms, and clearly stated. If more than one problem is identified, agreement is reached as to which problem will be addressed. A problem may involve anything from a description of a person's current communication status to an analysis of a service delivery issue with a specific population.
- *Step 2: Investigate and explore the issues relevant to the problem.* The problem is analysed and different reasons for the problem explored. Students are encouraged to draw on past knowledge to understand the problem and identify key themes/issues.
- *Step 3: Identify a range of solutions to the problem.* Solutions for change are then generated. All possible solutions are put forward for moving from the current state to the desired state, identifying the advantages and disadvantages of each.
- *Step 4: Identify areas of further investigation.* Students are required to identify the gaps in the knowledge available to them and what additional information is required in order to select between the different options. The best solution is selected and the rationale for why the choice was made is made explicit.
- *Step 5: Agree areas for investigation and an action plan.* As a group, the students then agree a list of terminology, topics and issues to be investigated; discuss how these investigations might be achieved; and decide on an action plan, detailing methods to be used.
- *Step 6: Independent investigation.* The students seek the information to meet the aims independently. This may take the form of further group meetings or be undertaken individually.
- *Step 7: Share outcomes of investigations.* Results are then pooled and information shared as to the sources of information used. The problem is revisited in light of new information and any new gaps identified for further investigation.
- *Step 8: Choose a solution and justify.* The best solution is selected and the rationale for why the choice was made is made explicit. The students are also encouraged to reflect on the learning achieved and consider its relevance.

The decision process is involved at all stages of the course, starting with a specified problem framework in the earlier years and then applied, in the later years, to a range of contexts that encourage adaptation and generalization.

Problem framework

The problem framework is unique to the case-based approach and involves a seven-stage process (see Figure 2.1) applied to individual real-life cases. Each stage is considered a problem to be solved, with the eight decision steps applied. Core language pathology modules covering disorders of articulation, phonology, semantics, sentence processing and pragmatics are taught using two cases, a paediatric case and an adult case. These are introduced towards the end of the first year with the articulation cases, and delivered predominantly in the second year, with the exception of the pragmatic cases that occur in the third year. An example of the adult case in the sentence-processing module, Case AL (Webster and Whitworth, 2003; Lum et al., 2002), is used to illustrate the framework. Other modules, e.g. clinical education and audiology, apply the decision process but adapt the problem framework to the subject matter. An example of this is given in more detail later in the chapter. All work is carried out in small groups of between six and eight students. Group work is regularly reported back to the larger group to monitor decision making and discuss differences that emerge.

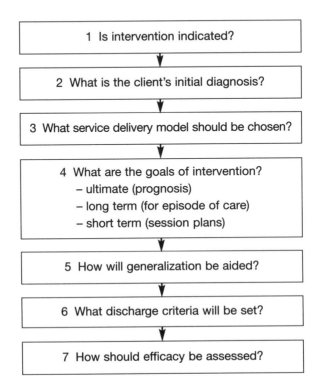

Figure 2.1 Problem framework based on Dodd (1995).

For the case of AL, students are provided with a short history (this could also be in the form of a referral letter) (see Figure 2.2) and a narrative sample.

Case AL: adult sentence processing

AL (66 years) is a retired electrical safety officer. He received 11 years of formal education, initially at school and then at various night school/training courses. He lives with his wife. Their two children live locally and visit regularly with their grandchildren. Hobbies include indoor/outdoor bowls, gardening and caravanning. He enjoys quizzes and bingo at the Speech after Stroke club, and has a very active social life.

He suffered a CVA 10 years ago while on holiday, leaving him with severe dysphasia and right hemiparesis (particularly in the lower limb). He received a small amount of speech and language therapy during his nine weeks in hospital, followed by community-based intervention for two years on discharge from hospital. He was then referred to a Speech after Stroke club, which he continues to attend. Although AL recognizes that his speech has improved dramatically since his CVA, he remains dissatisfied with the progress he has made.

Figure 2.2 Initial information given on case AL in stage 2.

Question 1. Is intervention indicated?

From this initial information and language sample, the group is required to develop a response as to whether or not intervention is indicated. This draws on the students' knowledge of what constitutes 'normal' communication, requiring them to consider the relationship between impairment, disability and social handicap, to reflect on potential for change and perceptions of the problem, and then to form an early hypothesis as to a possible diagnosis. In order to proceed to the next stage, the group is required to indicate what further information they would need to confirm or refute their tentative diagnosis. Requests for information must be specific (e.g. performance on a particular assessment).

Specifically, theoretical models of sentence processing, methods of analysing spontaneous speech samples, and candidacy and prognostic issues following neurological deficit are explored in an interactive teaching session. Students are required wherever possible to recall previous relevant knowledge and/or clinical experience to activate prior knowledge, a central tenet of PBL (Schmidt, 1993). The interactive nature of the classes and the constant drawing on past academic knowledge and clinical experiences foster this. Group work then follows, where students begin to formulate their hypotheses and identify areas for further investigation. Early in the module, students are encouraged to draw on a targeted reference list from which they are to input into group work. As the module progresses, students are required to explore and present back for class discussion complex issues in sentence processing that require greater self-directed learning. Providing early direction to the literature is supported by Dolmans and Schmidt (1996), who reported that students develop self-directed learning skills despite being guided in their decisions on what to read or explore further.

Question 2. What is AL's initial diagnosis?

In response to identifying areas where further information is needed, data from AL's initial assessment are given to each of the groups, and they then proceed with diagnosis. Assessment tools and methods used with sentence-processing impairments are explored here, again within an interactive teaching session, and linked with different theoretical positions. At this stage the students are required, within their groups, to identify the nature of the communication problem, address issues of severity, and highlight possible contributing causal and maintenance factors. Every decision must be supported by evidence or theoretical positions taken in the literature.

Question 3. What service delivery model should be chosen?

Before embarking on content of intervention, service delivery issues are explored for AL. Decisions as to who will be the agent of therapy (e.g. clinician, a family member, other professionals), whether individual or group therapy may be offered, the length and frequency of sessions (e.g. daily/weekly/fortnightly/monthly), the location of therapy (e.g. his home, clinic), the period of therapy contracted for, etc., are all considered here and the students are again required to justify all decisions made.

Question 4. What are the goals of intervention?

The students are then required to determine what specific aspects of communication should be targeted and plan an intervention programme for AL. Aims are specified with respect to: (a) ultimate goals (prognosis); and (b) long-term goals (for episode of care). Then, selecting one long-term goal, the students are required to apply a further framework for planning intervention. This involves setting short-term (sessional) goals and specifying the prerequisites necessary for achieving the goal, the underlying therapeutic approach, materials, hierarchies of difficulty, feedback and intended outcomes. Preparation for the casework involves both reviewing the literature for evidence-based interventions and planning therapy within a workshop session for a range of other sentence-level impairments. Theories of therapy are teased out at this stage as part of the group discussion.

Question 5. How will generalization be aided?

This approach assumes that generalization of target behaviour needs to be facilitated and will not usually carry over spontaneously into functional situations. The students are therefore required to propose explicitly how they might go about maximizing AL's potential for generalizing therapy targets into real-life circumstances, drawing on social models of therapy, and exploring issues of measurement and accountability. By this stage, the time spent in the small groups is much greater than that spent in the large group.

Question 6. What discharge criteria will be set?

Criteria for discharge are then set, considering possible reasons for discharge (e.g. target behaviour reached, progress not attributed to therapy, no progress or plateauing of progress), along with consideration given to AL's wishes, generalization, motivation, contextual factors and possibility of continued monitoring. The process of discharge (e.g. shared expectations, counselling) is also revisited.

Question 7. How should efficacy be assessed?

The final area involving efficacy explores not only the reasons for measuring the efficacy of therapy (e.g. accountability, revision of clinical decisions, work satisfaction, validity of improvement), but also possible experimental designs that will allow effectiveness to be measured in a clinically valid and useful way. The relationships between efficacy and earlier decisions of candidacy and goal setting are drawn out. This is carried out within both an interactive teaching session to draw on existing knowledge and within the groups.

The assessment of the module is based on a second case where the students are presented, again, with brief historical information, a written language sample and some selected assessment results. Each student is required to provide an individual written discussion using the problem framework for this case.

Evolution of the decision process

By the third year, students have established a firm grasp of the CBPS framework and it is possible to embed particular aspects of the framework within more varied teaching styles and to apply knowledge to more complex cases.

An example of this is seen in the audiology module. Two cases are presented in class from the perspective of an audiologist who focuses on diagnosis and treatment. One is an adult with acquired hearing impairment, the other a child with a profound congenital loss. Students are required to read about specified topics and to solve particular problems, in groups, outside class time, and there are lectures on specific techniques. In addition to this case-based work, invited speakers present two-hour seminars: a parent of a hearing impaired child; a teacher specializing in hearing impairment; a specialist speech and language therapist; and a teacher of sign language. There is also a debate on a controversial issue related to hearing impairment, e.g. 'Should parents have the right to consent to cochlear implantation of their young children?', in which students play roles (e.g. surgeon, representatives of the hearing-impaired community, sign language supporter, teacher). The information provided during the course is then assessed using a case-based approach. An example of an assessment for this module is set out in Figure 2.3.

Assessment: audiology module

You are a newly appointed speech and language therapist (SLT). The senior SLT has sent you the following letter. Your task is to respond to her requests.

Dear Monica,
I enclose a photocopy of the ENT notes on Sophie Benton. I have had several enquiries about Sophie in the last few weeks, concerning her hearing and communication skills. It would be very useful if you would compile a report that summarizes the results of her hearing assessments (including relevance and interpretation of all tests), and whether the hearing aids are likely to be benefiting her.

I also enclose a note from Mary Parsons, teacher of the deaf who visits Sophie at Newmills School, asking for our opinion on whether Sophie's speech and language problems can be explained by her hearing impairment, or whether she has an additional communication impairment. Could you please follow this through. If this is not clear from the notes, would you advise Mary which other investigations might be needed.

Many thanks,
Judy Crozier, Senior Speech and Language Therapist

The photocopied ENT notes consist of reports and letters spanning three years of Sophie's care. Audiological test results are presented using a range of different techniques.

Figure 2.3 Example of assessment for the audiology module in stage 3.

The clinical curriculum

The clinical curriculum is designed to complement the problem-based approach in the academic modules, reinforcing the seven-stage case framework in the early placements and promoting problem solving in wider contexts as the student nears graduation. Specific developments within the curriculum include the following.

Early campus-based placements

To ensure students have both a clear grasp of the approach and practice at applying the framework in a clinical context, the first two placements, offered in the second year of the course, take place on campus under the supervision of university clinical staff. A paediatric clinic and an aphasia clinic provide exposure to both child and adult cases, and the case-based framework provides the key scaffold for approaching individual case management. This is reinforced by university clinicians focused on this approach. With the move off campus in the final two years, a number of other strategies are in place to facilitate the approach being used in clinics within the broader community.

Supervisory training in PBL and CBPS

While the broadest of strategies is the fostering of a partnership between the higher education institution and service providers, where the education of speech and language therapists is considered a joint responsibility, ongoing targeted input into the community is essential. A key focus of this strategy is the provision of regular supervisory training offered at introductory and advanced levels. This training is well attended; supervisors who have not attended at least to the introductory level are the exception. Training at introductory level includes an introduction to PBL and its application to the clinical setting, including the case-based problem framework, while advanced-level courses identify key components of the process and expand on these.

A reflective model of supervision (Mandy, 1989) is encouraged with supervisors (on and off campus) and also introduced to the students. This model aims to encourage a deep approach to learning and provides a structured framework that engages the student in reflective learning within the clinical setting. An essential part of this process is allowing both the student and supervisor time to analyse and reflect on clinical experiences prior to coming together to discuss the experience. The success of supervisors adopting this approach is tied in closely to acknowledging the changed role and focus of the clinical supervisor from 'expert clinician' to 'facilitator'. This is addressed through such topics as direct and indirect teaching styles, structuring feedback sessions to increase the focus on the student reporting, and keeping educational philosophy at the forefront.

Professional contexts clinical placement

A further strategy has been the introduction of a professional contexts placement for final year students. This placement can take place in either a campus- or community-based clinic and involves the student focusing on a service-delivery problem in addition to managing a small caseload. The student is required to apply his or her problem-solving skills to an issue of a service-delivery nature, and complete whatever research or activity is required to solve the problem. This is then written up as a report for a specified and real target audience and presented to the clinic involved. Examples of these clinics have included:

- an evaluation of discharge pathways for adult neurology services
- examination of the effectiveness of intensive speech and language therapy as a service delivery model for people with aphasia
- evaluation of parental and professional satisfaction of early intervention for children with pre-school special needs
- evaluation of phonological awareness groups
- comparison of home/clinic/school-based therapy for specific paediatric cases
- evaluation of one method of delivering a signing system to staff working with adults with autism and hearing impairment
- evaluation of parental involvement and decision making in gastrostomy.

Competency-based assessment framework

The development of a competency-based assessment format that is structured loosely around the case framework is the final strategy for integrating our CBPS approach, allowing transparency between what is required in clinic and how the student is assessed. This assessment format remains the same throughout the course with the student moving along a continuum from absence of competency to emerging competency to acknowledged competency. Where necessary, the assessment is supplemented by additional specific competencies, e.g. as in the case of the professional contexts placement, which may not fit specifically into the case framework but expand on other problem-solving skills.

Issues in implementing the PBL approach

Making groups work

Effective group working is fundamental to good PBL. Where group work constitutes a substantial part of students' learning, and even assessment, it is common for students to focus on issues such as 'are the groups fair?', 'does every group member take an equal share in the work?', 'do the groups have students of equal ability?' and 'are there clashes of personality?'. For the group to work effectively, it is necessary for each of the members to take responsibility for recognizing and solving potential difficulties that may occur in the dynamics of the group. When this operates successfully, it is a powerful learning experience for cooperative and mature working.

Over time, we have developed a number of strategies to facilitate effective group working. As part of the admissions procedure, the applicants are placed in groups and asked to solve a problem rather than being given formal interviews. The intention is to select students who will both benefit from our particular approach to teaching and learning and be willing to engage in this learning style (good performance in the PBL task will also reveal the kind of interpersonal skills that will make good clinicians). In the first year, as part of the clinical education strand, students take part in team-building workshops to enhance their ability to take an active role in a group interaction while being encouraging to others.

There are also important practical considerations. The number of students in each group should be large enough that there is a good spread of experience and ability brought to bear in the work, but not so large that individuals never get a chance to contribute. Groups of between six and eight students have been found to work well. It has also been important to both randomly assign groups and change the groups as often as possible (usually each semester). Students will often ask to self-select group members, which, given the tendency for people of similar abilities and enthusiasms to stay together, can result in skewed groups. Given the students' busy timetables, it has been important when randomly assigning members that each group has time when it can work together outside classes. In the second year, the same group of students is assigned to a CBPS group as to a clinic placement group in order that they have the same free time; this has increased satisfaction with group working.

Finally, there are rules about how each group session operates, namely that one person 'scribes' and one person 'chairs'. The scribe is responsible for writing down everything said on a flipchart. This is important for the learning process in that the process of reaching a decision is mapped as well as the decision itself, and the group can see and agree that the process is being recorded accurately. The tutor will also have a record of the group's work. This is essential in a situation where we have insufficient tutors for each groups to be observed at all times (usually two tutors oversee six groups). The chair ensures that the group keeps on course and that everyone contributes. While groups working partially alone without a staff tutor have arisen predominantly from limited resources, Steele et al. (2000) found no difference in student performance on objective examinations following working in groups that were either peer- or staff-led. Steele et al. did report, however, that the students took more short cuts when working in a student-facilitated group, clearly a factor that both students and staff need to remain aware of. Given the essential role of the group in PBL, Hak and Maguire (2000) suggest that the cognitive activities of the group and how they are managed warrant more detailed description and analysis in future research.

Since the key principle of PBL is active learning, it is important that the students should understand why they are participating in this method of learning, and in particular, in our programme, why they are doing a hybrid version. This is made explicit in both teaching and documentation and, as far as possible, the same approach is encountered in their clinical practice. It is also stressed that collaborative working (for example, the shared management of clients) is an important competency when working as a speech and language therapist, and that group working gives them important clinical skills. This is reinforced in their second-year adult placement where the students collaborate to provide intensive treatment for clients with aphasia.

The role of the tutor

The role of the tutor in PBL is quite different from that of the traditional teacher and this is carried over to the CBPS groups. Tutors must not see themselves as the expert who is there to tell the students 'the answer' at the end of the process. This would undermine the active learning of the students that must be seen as equal in value to that of the tutors. It is also necessary for the tutor to suppress an often-natural desire to share his or her (usually) greater experience with the students, keeping in mind the limits of passive learning. The ways in which tutors intervene in sessions and give feedback are, therefore, critical to the process. When a tutor is observing a group session they should not intervene, except when asked for clarification or perhaps where the group dynamic is a serious problem. Students may get feedback by presenting the outcome of sessions to each other, and discussing any differences that arise. The tutor might summarize outcomes across the different groups and give alternative interpretations (although these should not be presented as 'better' outcomes). Written summary feedback may also be given. The tutor, or staff facilitator, must therefore believe in the efficacy of the process; groups may appear to go in a very tangential direction in a session but almost always work it out in the end. Dolmans et al. (2001) warn also of the tendency for tutors, when their own satisfaction wanes, to revert back to previous methods of delivery, such as teacher-directed models. Tutors, when faced with groups that may not be operating effectively, 'should hold onto the philosophy of student-directed learning' (Dolmans et al., 2001: 885) and be guided constantly by this.

All group facilitators involved in the University of Newcastle speech and language therapy programme have expert knowledge. It is not, however, a requirement that this be the case in a pure PBL programme and the possibility of employing additional tutorial support may be explored in the future. There is some evidence to suggest that group facilitators who have content knowledge, as opposed to no expert knowledge, do influence the tutoring process in such a way that improves the performance of the group and facilitates subsequent self-directed learning (Schmidt et al., 1993; Hay and Katsikitis, 2001). De Grave et al. (1999), however, explored students' perceptions of tutor characteristics and found that, while students perceive tutors to be most effective if they have both expert knowledge and can focus on the learning process, it was more important for the tutor to be able to guide the learning process than to be familiar with the problem content.

Types of problem to be used

The majority of our problems revolve around real cases, a factor that has been shown to enhance student satisfaction with PBL (Aspegren et al., 1998; Dammers et al., 2001). While it would be possible to use manufactured 'pure' cases, real-life cases have two primary advantages. First, from early in their education, students deal with the complexities of imperfect assessment data. Second, the students learn about the whole person, taking into consideration the communicative, social and psychological needs of the individual in all treatment decisions. Each case presented has undergone a management programme so that the students, after making their own management decisions, can be informed of the real-life outcome. Giving positive examples of efficacious treatment is highly motivating for the students.

Since students need to make use of the decision process and problem framework when encountering all potential clients, they work on a range of cases. The assessment cases are therefore not replications of the cases worked on during the module. Using the tutor's own cases is advantageous, since the assessments carried out on the client will then map onto the theoretical models used in teaching, and the relationship between theory and practice will be highly explicit. The cases have been shown to work best if the students are only given a minimal amount of information about the clients' communication and are required to think about and request which assessments they would like completed. The students are then making active decisions about how they would assess the client, mimicking the clinical situation.

Evaluation of the CBPS approach at Newcastle University

An important characteristic of the hybrid PBL model we use is the structure given to the work the students do that revolves around the seven steps of case management. This unusually structured approach has both advantages and disadvantages. The benefits of the model are reflected in the reasons for adopting the case management structure into our curriculum. The first is a practical one. As students have a limited amount of time to devote to the group working and self-study of the CBPS modules, we need to direct this time and make it maximally useful. Second, the case management steps give a structure that can be applied to every case, whether it is in class or in clinic. It is therefore anticipated that theory and practice will be integrated throughout the academic and clinical streams. Third, the seven steps ensure that the language pathology modules give as much time to learning about therapy as about assessment. In more traditional lecture courses, there has been a tendency to give greater emphasis to assessment and diagnosis. Fourth, the CBPS approach gives students experience of discussing cases together in a way which will enhance case sharing and multiprofessional working as speech and language therapists. Finally, the approach has many of the benefits of using a pure PBL approach. The students take responsibility for aspects of their own and their colleagues' learning. They learn to apply knowledge they already have and they develop an ability to find out information for themselves.

What are the drawbacks of the hybrid approach? Owing to the greater number of constraints than are seen within pure PBL curricula, there is necessarily a reduction in the amount of self-directed learning. Input is higher than on pure PBL courses and the attention of the students is drawn to targeted references. While a tension exists between allowing students to find appropriate library material themselves (which may then be inaccessible to the other students) and giving them reading lists so material can be, for example, put on short or reserved loan in the library, the latter decision is often taken. The modules are also structured in such a way that the same tutor gives lectures, conducts workshops and supervises group sessions for an individual case; this can make it difficult for the tutor to lose their role as 'expert' for the problem-based work. The way in which feedback during the group sessions is handled by the tutor is therefore especially important. Early in its implementation we also found that using the same structure can be repetitive for the students, with aspects becoming less challenging. To combat this, students in the second year are now encouraged to explore topics of their own interest for group discussion, and the third-year work has a wholly more diverse structure. Dolmans et al.'s (2001) earlier warning to tutors not to slip back into more traditional habits has also remained a priority as we have realized that course leaders need to work together to ensure that this does not happen. Team teaching, regular planned discussions between staff and annual away-days with outside speakers are strategies in place to monitor this.

To date, the feedback from students obtained in annual written assessments of all academic and clinical modules, and structured meetings to focus on CBPS specifically, has been highly positive. Students report, for example, strong links between theory and clinical practice, confidence in making diagnoses and planning appropriate intervention, and high motivation levels with the group learning process. Their input expressing dissatisfaction with CBPS has been heavily drawn on during the implementation of the approach, e.g. varying the format and assessment approach as exposure to the framework increases, grouping students on the basis of common clinical schedules, responding to unequal group contributions through the introduction of team building and assertiveness training. Some persistent negative responses continue to present, such as requests for more lecture time, less self-directed study and less group working; these are dealt with through continual efforts to make the pedagogical aims of the course explicit.

Specific measures are clearly needed to evaluate our CBPS approach to teaching the discipline of speech and language pathology. Previous research from both pure and hybrid models indicates that the benefits of PBL, as opposed to traditional teaching, include continued learning after graduation, better retention of knowledge and greater patient satisfaction from services received from healthcare professionals educated in a PBL context (Lewis et al., 1992). The systematic evaluation of courses is, however, highly complex. While a small significant effect found in a review of controlled evaluation studies did seem to demonstrate evidence of effectiveness (Smits et al., 2002), identifying true outcome measures and quantifying these remain a challenge. Although other speech and language pathology courses have adopted a PBL approach to education (in Australia, Hong Kong and Scandinavia), as yet there are no published research reports evaluating the outcome of these courses.

We are in the process of evaluating the PBL approach used in the education of speech and language therapists at the University of Newcastle. Four specific measures are being employed in this process.

1 Comparison of performance of students from the earlier non-PBL course with students on the revised course at graduation by comparing common assessments across the two courses (e.g. dissertation, speech and language pathology examination papers).
2 Measurement of student and employer satisfaction for the last three years of the old curricula to enable comparisons to be made with graduates of the new course as they enter the workforce.
3 Structured interviews with all staff and a range of clinical supervisors to evaluate the implementation of the course, to identify course revisions needed, and to gauge their opinions of the process of implementation and development of the new curricula.
4 Comparison of student evaluations of subjects taught in the new curriculum with evaluations of courses from the old curricula.

Until these data are collected and analysed, objective evaluation of our hybrid case-based, problem-solving approach to educating speech and language therapists cannot be provided. Anecdotal evidence to date, from both university and community clinicians, is highly supportive of qualitative changes in the nature of the student speech and language therapist at each stage of the course, and early analysis of clinical performance data suggests higher numbers of students both achieving distinction in their clinical placements and demonstrating greater attention to issues of self-evaluation and broader clinical contexts during examinations. In addition to evaluation, future issues for the course are the development of suitable assessment methods for assessing student performance, taking forward the areas of peer and self-assessment, and continuing to pursue the role of professional competence both in the curriculum and in the methods we use to teach it. And, finally, an ongoing feature of our activity will be to continually remind ourselves of the underlying educational philosophy we sought to adopt and avoid the path of least resistance by reverting back to our 'expert' roles and more didactic teaching.

Acknowledgements

The authors wish to acknowledge the clinical community of the North of England for their input and support, and all staff on the Speech and Language Sciences programme at Newcastle University for their persistent efforts and receptiveness to change.

References

Albanese M (2000) Problem-based learning: why curricula are likely to show little effect on knowledge and clinical skills. Medical Education 34: 729–738.

Albanese MA, Mitchell S (1993) Problem-based learning: a review of literature on its outcomes and implementation issues. Academic Medicine 68: 52–81.

Armstrong EG (1991) A hybrid model of problem-based learning. In Boud D, Feletti G (eds) The Challenge of Problem Based Learning. London: Kogan Page.

Aspegren K, Blomqvist P, Borgstrom A (1998) Live patients and problem-based learning. Medical Teacher 20: 417–420.

Biley FC, Smith KL (1999) Making sense of problem-based learning: the perceptions and experiences of undergraduate nursing students. Journal of Advanced Nursing 30: 1205–1212.

Bligh J, Lloyd-Jones G, Smith G (2000) Early effects of a new problem-based clinically oriented curriculum on students' perceptions of teaching. Medical Education 34: 487–489.

Boud D, Feletti G (1991) The Challenge of Problem Based Learning. London: Kogan Page.

Bovee ML, Gran DF (2000) Comparison of two teaching methods in a chiropractic clinical science course. Journal of Allied Health 29: 157–160.

Brandon JE, Majumdar B (1997) An introduction and evaluation of problem-based learning in health professions education. Family & Community Health 20: 1–15.

Colliver JA (2000) Effectiveness of problem-based learning curricula: research and theory. Academic Medicine 75: 259–266.

Dalton S (1999) Problem-based learning: a method that encourages critical thinking. Health Care Food and Nutrition Focus 15(9): 4–6.

Dammers J, Spence J, Thomas M (2001) Using real patients in problem-based learning: students' comments on the value of using real, as opposed to paper cases, in a problem-based learning module in general practice. Medical Education 35: 27–34.

de Grave W, Dolmans DH, van der Vleuten CP (1999) Profiles of effective tutors in problem-based learning: scaffolding student learning. Medical Education 33: 901–906.

de Virgilio G (1993) Problem-based learning for training primary health care managers in developing countries. Medical Education 27: 266–273.

Dodd BJ (1995) Differential diagnosis and treatment of speech disordered children. London: Whurr.

Dolmans DH, Gijselaers WH, Schmidt HG, van der Meer SB (1993) Problem effectiveness in a course using problem-based learning. Academic Medicine 68: 2107–2113.

Dolmans D, Schmidt HG (1996) The advantages of problem-based curricula. Postgraduate Medical Journal 72: 535–538.

Dolmans DH, Wolfhagen IH, van der Vleuten CP, Wijnen WH (2001) Solving problems with group work in problem-based learning: hold on to the philosophy. Medical Education 35: 884–889.

Dowd SB, Davidhizar R (1999) Using case studies to teach clinical problem-solving. Nurse Education 24(5): 42–46.

Fincham AG, Shuler CF (2001) The changing face of dental education: the impact of PBL. Journal of Dental Education 65: 406–421.

Hak T, Maguire P (2000) Group process: the black box of studies on problem-based learning. Academic Medicine 75: 769–772.

Hammel J, Royeen CB, Bagatell N, Chandler B, Jensen G, Loveland J, Stone G (1999) Student perspectives on problem-based learning in an occupational therapy curriculum: a multiyear qualitative evaluation. American Journal of Occupational Therapy 53: 199–206.

Hay PJ, Katsikitis M (2001) The 'expert' in problem-based and case-based learning: necessary or not? Medical Education 35: 22–26.

Houlden R., Collier CP, Frid PJ, John SL, Pross H (2001) Problems identified by tutors in a hybrid problem-based learning curriculum. Academic Medicine 76: 81.

Huey D (2001) The potential utility of problem-based learning in the education of clinical psychologists and others. Education for Health 14: 11–19.

Lewis ME, Buckley A, Kong M, Mellsop GW (1992) Innovation and change. Annals of Community-Oriented Education 5: 193–198.

Lum C, Cox R, Kilgour J (2002) Universities of Sussex and Edinburgh. PATSy: a database of clinical cases for teaching and research. Retrieved from http://www.patsy.ac.uk

Mandy S (1989) Facilitating student learning in clinical education. Australian Journal of Human Communication Disorders 6: 83–93.

Margetson DB (1999) The relation between understanding and practice in problem-based medical education. Medical Education 33: 359–364.

Maudsley G (1999) Do we all mean the same thing by 'problem-based learning'? A review of the concepts and a formulation of the ground rules. Academic Medicine 74: 178–185

Miller AP, Schwartz PL, Loten EG (2000) 'Systems integration': a middle way between problem-based learning and traditional courses. Medical Teacher 22: 51–58.

Nandi PL, Chan JN, Chan CP, Chan P, Chan LP (2000) Undergraduate medical education: comparison of problem-based learning and conventional teaching. Hong Kong Medical Journal 6: 301–306.

Neufeld VR, Barrows HS (1974) The 'McMaster philosophy': an approach to medical education. Journal of Medical Education 49: 1040–1050.

Neufeld VR, Woodward CA, MacLeod SM (1989) The McMaster MD program: a case study of renewal in medical education. Academic Medicine 64: 423–432.

Ozuah PO, Curtis J, Stein RE (2001) Impact of problem-based learning on residents' self-directed learning. Archives of Pediatrics & Adolescent Medicine 155: 669–672.

Sable MR, Larrive LS, Gayer D (2001) Problem-based learning: opportunities and barriers for training interdisciplinary health care teams. Journal of Teaching in Social Work 21: 217–234.

Sadlo G (1997) Problem-based learning enhances the education experiences of occupational therapy students. Education for Health 10: 101–114.

Schmidt HG (1993) Foundations of problem-based learning: some explanatory notes. Medical Education 27: 422–432.

Smits PBA, Verbeek JHAM, de Buisonje CD (2002) Problem based learning in continuing medical education: a review of controlled evaluation studies. British Medical Journal 324: 153–156.

Steele DJ, Medder JD, Turner P (2000) A comparison of learning outcomes and attitudes in student- versus faculty-led problem-based learning: an experimental study. Medical Education 34: 23–29.

Verhoeven BH, Verwijnen GM, Scherpbier AJJA, Holdrinet RSG, Oeseburg B, Bulte JA, van der Vleuten CPM (1998) Medical Teacher 20: 310–316.

Webster J, Whitworth A (2003) AL: accessing the predicate argument structure. In Byng S, Swinburn K, Pound C (eds) Aphasia Therapy File, vol 2. Hove, East Sussex: Psychology Press (in press).

Chapter 3
Peer placements

KIM GRUNDY

Introduction

Peer placements have been running at De Montfort University, Leicester, since their effectiveness was evaluated through pilot studies in 1994 (Grundy, 1994). They were initially introduced as a potential solution to the nationally experienced shortage of clinical placements – if two students went on a placement normally allocated to one student, then only half the number of placements would be needed. It was soon found that providing a solution to the numbers problem was by no means the only benefit of peer placements.

This chapter briefly outlines Kolb's (1984) model of experiential learning and relates this to clinical placement learning. It goes on to outline a model of peer placements and consider how the peering of students may facilitate experiential learning. It then reports on feedback from students and clinical teachers on the peer placement experience and discusses the development of peer placements into peer tutoring placements.

Kolb's theory of experiential learning

Basing his work on that of John Dewey, Kurt Lewin and Jean Piaget, Kolb (1984) put forward a detailed model of adult learning termed *experiential learning*. Kolb offers a working definition of (experiential) learning as '... the process whereby knowledge is created through the transformation of experience' (Kolb, 1984: 38). He presents his model in the form of a cycle (Figure 3.1). First the learner has an experience (experience) during which he or she observes and then reflects (reflection), he or she then reviews the experience in relation to his or her current knowledge (conceptualization) and then acts on the basis of this reviewed knowledge (experimentation). This final step provides the learner with a new experience and the cycle repeats.

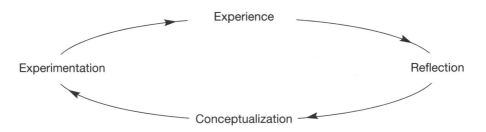

Figure 3.1 Kolb's (1984) experiential learning cycle.

Within the model it is important to appreciate that there is duality in the meaning of the term 'experience'. Experience is both subjective and objective. Subjectively, experience includes personal feelings and thoughts within the situation including those arising through previous experience, beliefs and knowledge. Objectively, experience relates to the reality of what is happening. Through this acknowledgement of the duality of experience it becomes clear that no learner enters a learning situation as a 'blank slate'. Each of us enters any experience having had many previous experiences that leave us with beliefs, expectations and modes of response in relation to the upcoming experience.

To exemplify this in relation to clinical experience, we might consider a student observing a clinician taking a case history. During this observation the student may simply be observing what is happening and taking notes for later reflection. Alternatively, the student may be *reflecting-in-action* (Schon, 1987), that is comparing what is observed with, for example, previous experiences of the case-taking process or previous knowledge/beliefs regarding that particular client group. After the event, the student will engage in *reflection-on-action* (Schon, 1987), that is the student will review the experience and consider how his or her previous knowledge/beliefs/feelings fit with this new experience. The process of accommodating previously held knowledge/beliefs/feelings to adapt to this new experience is the stage of conceptualization in Kolb's model. After this, the student will have his or her own turn at taking a case history. His or her actions during this experience will derive from his or her process of conceptualization and he or she will try out behaviours based on the resultant knowledge/beliefs/feelings. As such, the student will have a new experience and the cycle will begin again.

Now the cycle involves the student in direct experience. The student is likely to observe and reflect during the experience (reflection-in-action). For example, he or she may observe that the client is repeatedly responding with yes/no answers. Reflection may (or may not) cause the student to identify that he or she is asking closed questions. At this point, the student may move straight into active experimentation and begin to ask open questions. This will provide a new experience for reflection: the strategy will work or it will not. After the event, the student may reflect-on-action and may then evaluate previously held views on open and closed questions (conceptualization). The results of this evaluation will affect the way in which the student asks questions of clients in future case-history taking sessions (experimentation), providing a new experience for the cycle to repeat.

What is a peer placement?

Quite simply, a peer placement involves two students participating together in a placement that would traditionally be allocated to one student. Both students take part together in the activities that one student would have engaged in, so there are no additional resources required in terms of clinical teachers or clients.

What is the aim of a peer placement?

The aim of any clinical placement is for students to learn. The specifics of what the students are intended to learn on any particular placement will be agreed between the university and the host organization but, whatever the specifics, students will be expected to develop their current knowledge and skills and to acquire new knowledge and skills. The aim of a peer placement is to facilitate this learning.

How does a peer placement work?

Below is a model of how a peer placement can work in a community clinic, hospital outpatient department or other settings where clinicians are working directly with clients. The roles of students and clinical teacher change as students gain experience and become more independent in clinical work. (Two fictitious students have been used for exemplification.) There are three stages to the model, the first of which is the observation stage, where both students are engaged in observation of their clinical teacher. This is followed by the interim stage, where each student observes the other with their clinical teacher present, and the final stage, where each student observes the other without observation from their clinical teacher. The length of each stage will depend on the nature and length of the placement and the perceived abilities of the students.

Observation period

It is generally accepted that students need an opportunity to observe clinicians in practice before being expected to intervene with clients themselves. Some placements are purely observational and students would not move beyond this stage if engaged on an observation placement. It is important to recognize that students can continue to learn from observation of experienced clinicians throughout (and beyond) their student life and, even when they have moved on to the interim and final stages of the model, will still benefit from opportunities to observe their clinician.

Treatment session 1

• Martha and Rose observe their clinical teacher working with client 1. (If this is not possible, Martha observes the clinical teacher working with client 1 and Rose looks at case notes for client 2.)

Treatment session 2

• Martha and Rose observe their clinical teacher working with client 2. (If this is not possible, Rose observes the clinical teacher working with client 2 and Martha looks at case notes for client 1.)

Treatment session 3

• The clinical teacher works with client 3.
• Martha and Rose discuss their observations of clients 1 and 2 together, shape them for presentation to their clinical teacher and identify questions for their clinical teacher. Once they have enough experience they will also formulate the next step for intervention for both clients.

Post-treatment session

• Students relay their discussions to their clinical teacher.

Interim period

At this stage the students are beginning to work with clients under the close supervision of their clinical teacher. Again, the number of sessions worked in this way will depend on the nature of the placement, the client group and the students' development of skills.

Treatment session 1

• The clinical teacher and Rose observe Martha working with client 1.

Treatment session 2

• The clinical teacher and Martha observe Rose working with client 2.

Treatment session 3

• The clinical teacher works with client 3.
• Martha relays to Rose her experience of the treatment session with client 1; Rose then gives Martha her observations of the session.

- Rose relays to Martha her experience of the treatment session with client 2; Martha then gives Rose her observations of the session.
- Both students formulate feedback and questions for their clinical teacher and plan the next treatment sessions for their clients.

Post-treatment session

- Rose and Martha feed back to the clinical teacher.
- The clinical teacher feeds back to the students.

Final stage

At this stage the students are beginning to work more independently. Instead of being observed by their clinical teacher, they work together, observe one another and feed back their experiences to their clinical teacher after the intervention sessions.

Treatment session 1

- Martha works with client 1, Rose observes.
- The clinical teacher works with another client, or carries out other work.

Treatment session 2

- Rose works with client 2, Martha observes.
- The clinical teacher works with another client, or carries out other work.

Treatment session 3

- Rose and Martha observe the clinical teacher working with client 3.

Post-treatment session

- Rose and Martha feed back their experiences and observations to one another, and the clinical teacher facilitates discussion.
- Rose and Martha plan the next sessions for their clients.

It is particularly in this final stage that a major benefit of peer placements to the clinical teacher can be seen. The students are working independently, allowing the clinical teacher to see additional clients or catch up on other work.

Peer placements and experiential learning theory

To state the obvious, at any stage in the model of peer placements there are two students rather than one, which means that for any given experience, two unique sets of knowledge/beliefs/feelings are brought to bear. At the observation stage, students are expected to reflect on the experience together. It is likely that their different prior conceptualizations will allow them to expand their observations, answer questions for one another, identify mutual areas of confusion and facilitate the formulation of clear and specific questions for their clinical teacher.

At the interim stage, there are three people engaged in the learning cycle: the active student, the observing student and the clinical teacher. Each one brings to the experience his or her own unique conceptualizations. Following the experience, each one reflects. The active student has reflection-in-action to bring to the discussion, whereas the observing student perhaps has an additional perspective of more objective observation. Their discussion may engender more enhanced conceptualization and plans for future experimentation than the cogitations of one student alone. The clinical teacher brings to the feedback session a greater wealth of experience than either student and can further enhance conceptualization and plans for experimentation.

At the final stage, the peer students' discussion is likely to benefit from their previous experiences of peer feedback sessions and they are likely to be fully conversant with conceptualizing and planning for experimentation together. In addition, given that their clinical teacher has not observed their sessions, they will need to develop strategies for effectively feeding back their observations, interpretations and future plans.

Best and Rose (1996) consider Kolb's learning theory in relation to clinical education and suggest that the cycle allows for the thorough integration of theory and practice. These authors also discuss collaborative learning (paired clinical placements) and suggest that the collaborative model provides students with: 'peer support in a new and stressful situation; peer review in a non-threatening relationship and opportunities to develop relevant professional skills related to teamwork and communication and to promote learner independence' (Best and Rose, 1996: 120). Lincoln et al. (1996) hypothesize that peer learning may have the benefits of broadening perspectives, developing professional interaction skills and promoting professional socialization.

The student experience of peer placements

Peer placements have proved to be very popular with students. The placement mode for the pilot studies was block placement of four or five weeks' duration that often required students to move to an unknown part of the country and live in 'digs' or nurses' accommodation. Written feedback was obtained from the 16 students who participated in the pilot studies, which asked them to compare the peer experience with their previous experience of singleton placements. They reported:

- greater emotional and academic security resulting in increased confidence, improved problem solving, less homesickness, less pressure and reduced panic
- having attended lectures together they could 'translate' clinicians' terminology or 'spark off' memories from lectures or reading for each other
- having 'checked out' with each other that neither of them knew something they felt more confident to ask questions
- the observing student could note things the other might miss or forget and could look for specific things, such as timing and attention
- they could help each other out in sessions – for example while getting used to conducting assessments, one student could carry out the procedure while the other recorded the results
- their observation skills improved through peer observation
- their different perspectives broadened their knowledge
- they could learn from each other
- they could take on more clients between them than if they were alone, resulting in a broader range of client experience
- two students provided opportunities for small group work
- their peer discussion resulted in more dynamic interaction with clinicians
- they found that feedback from their peer related specifically to what they were aiming to achieve and was positive
- they found it easier to take criticism from their peer than their clinician
- feelings of competition could be motivating
- they felt less pressure to do *everything* correctly
- it was easier to talk to other professionals when with a peer
- their session plans were more thoroughly thought through
- they developed their team-working skills.

It would appear that the hypothesized benefits in relation to the experiential learning model are supported by this feedback. Students' acknowledgment of better problem solving and the broadening of knowledge through their different perspectives suggests that the peer experience did indeed facilitate conceptualization. They also indicated more dynamic interactions with clinical teachers and more thoroughly thought through session plans, which would seem to support the expectation that conceptualization and experimentation would be improved in a peer placement. As anticipated by Best and Rose (1996), students reported stress reduction through attending placement with a peer. Students' statements that it was easier to talk to other professionals and that their team-working skills improved would seem to support the expectation of improvement in professional teamwork and communication skills (Best and Rose, 1996), and professional socialization and interaction skills (Lincoln et al., 1996).

McAllister (1996) points out that, increasingly, health professionals are required to work as part of a team and that a key mode of learning for those working in health-related professions is through peer learning. She suggests that it should be a goal of clinical education to establish the process of peer learning. McAllister also refers to research that establishes the economic benefits of peer placements: 'Ladyshewsky and Healey (1990), in a Canadian study of physiotherapy students, reported greater efficiency in the planning and orientation phases of students' placements, greater input into problem-solving and more time available for improving the quality of client care. Perhaps more importantly for clinic administrators ... two senior students were able to carry a caseload greater than that of a solo clinician. This finding has recently been replicated with a study by Ladyshewsky and Barrie (1996) with speech therapy students in Australia' (McAllister, 1996: 20).

The clinical teacher experience of peer placements

The feedback from clinical teachers on peer placements has also been positive. Indeed, after experiencing a peer placement, some clinical teachers will only take students in pairs. The 14 clinical teachers involved in the pilot studies were also asked to provide written feedback on the peer experience compared with the singleton experience. They reported:

- peer discussions away from the clinician allowed for brainstorming and enabled students to clarify their thinking; questions resulting from peer discussions were therefore clear and specific
- students were better at problem solving and less dependent on their clinical teachers
- peer discussion with the clinician present enabled the clinician to join in and take the students further; discussions were therefore more dynamic
- in one setting, the clients joined in the discussion and gave students feedback. These clients were very positive about the peer placement
- students could be expected to find their own way around service locations and could take care of themselves during breaks
- there was a greatly reduced 'pastoral care' role for clinical teachers outside of clinic hours
- students could work more independently of their clinical teacher sooner than with singleton placements
- they felt more confident about leaving students with clients even early on in the placement
- students did not need to be with their clinical teacher as much as singleton students so there was more time for the clinical teacher to get on with other work
- they felt less pressure than when supervising one student.

The feedback from clinical teachers that problem solving improved, that peer discussion with the clinical teacher was more dynamic and that students could work more independently of their clinical teacher would seem to support the hypothesis that experiential learning is facilitated through peer placements.

As stated in the introduction to this chapter, peer placements were initially introduced as a solution to the general shortage of clinical placements. The pilot studies were carried out to establish whether or not they offered a workable solution to the numbers problem. Overall, the results of the pilot studies seemed to suggest that not only were peer placements a workable mode of placement but, in fact, seemed to offer an enhanced learning experience for students and a more satisfying teaching experience for clinicians. This finding provided motivation to continue to develop peer placements and seek solutions to those problems identified by the participants in the pilot studies.

Problems with peer placements identified by students, and their solutions

Below are the problems with peer placements identified by students who participated in the pilot studies. Each problem is followed by potential solutions that have evolved through subsequent experience.

- *Problem*: when at the final stage of observing each other without their clinical teacher present they worried that, as students, they were less likely to know (than their clinical teacher) if the methods that they were using were acceptable.
- *Solutions*: regular observation of students by the clinical teacher throughout the placement; regular discussion time with the clinical teacher before and after all intervention sessions.
- *Problem*: if students got different gradings (or marks) for their placement, then this could be difficult to accept.
- *Solutions*: preparation of students before they start the placement can help (see below). An alternative suggestion is to remove gradings or marks from peer placements and use a satisfactory/unsatisfactory evaluation with a profile of skills and areas for development for each student.
- *Problem*: some students felt that it was difficult to make an individual impression on clinical teachers whom they did not see very often. Efforts made by peers to make an individual impression occasionally led to unhelpful vying for attention. (What needs to be recognized here is that the students' concern is, at least partly, to do with their assessment. If they are unable to make an individual impression on their clinical teacher, how will they get a fair assessment? The solutions offered above are therefore relevant here.)

- *Solutions*: ensure adequate time to observe each student working and some individual feedback and discussion time for each student.
- *Problem*: students were concerned that they might not be getting enough individual observation and feedback from their clinical teacher.
- *Solutions*: this may be the case if the model is run exactly as stated above and in the final stage students only work together and report back to their clinical teacher. To ensure that students continue to benefit from clinical teacher feedback it is important that clinical teachers observe students regularly throughout the placement. It is also helpful to occasionally observe and feed back to each student without their peer present.
- *Problem*: students were worried that they might develop some of the less desirable practices of their peer.
- *Solutions*: as above, regular observation and feedback from the clinical teacher will prevent this happening.
- *Problem*: it was possible to 'clique' together on placement and not interact with other staff.
- *Solutions*: preparation of students before they embark on a peer placement can help here. Clinical teachers can help by introducing both peers to other staff members and arranging for students to work with, or find out information from, their colleagues.

Problems with peer placements identified by clinicians, and their solutions

Actual problems experienced by clinical teachers who participated in the pilot studies were, in fact, very few. The main difficulty was the practical one of finding physical space to accommodate two students. Again, solutions that have evolved through subsequent experience are outlined.

- *Problem*: finding space for students to have their peer discussions so that the clinical teacher could work with another client at the same time.
- *Solutions*: students have successfully conducted their discussions in a variety of locations, including staff rooms, resource centres, on-site accommodation, staff canteens and even their own cars. It is, of course, essential that they maintain client confidentiality but, providing this is adhered to, they do not necessarily need a private clinic room for their discussions.
- *Problem*: having rooms that are not big enough to accommodate clinical teacher, carer, client and two students.
- *Solutions*: work with one student at a time and ensure adequate time for students to feed back their experiences to each other.

Potential problems envisaged by clinicians and their solutions

As well as the problems identified by those involved in the pilot studies, there are other potential problems envisaged by those considering trying a peer placement (see also Best and Rose, 1996). Over the past few years, clinical teachers and students have found creative solutions to most potential problems.

- *Problem*: mismatch between students. This appears to be the primary concern of clinicians considering taking a peer placement. What if the two students do not get on? What if one has demonstrably better clinical skills than the other? What if one student is much more forthcoming than the other and dominates discussions?
- *Solutions*: actual experience has shown that there are far fewer of these types of problem than might be anticipated. Allowing students to select their own peers tends to mitigate against temperamental mismatch and can reduce potential difficulties where there is a mismatch in skills. It is unlikely that one student will be strong in every aspect of clinical work while the other is weak in every aspect. The strengths of each peer can be highlighted for the other to learn from. Where one student is more dominant in discussion, this can be addressed directly and students directed to facilitate each other's comments. Ensuring there is some time for individual feedback to the clinical teacher can also help with this problem. Thorough preparation of students prior to the start of the placement is very pertinent to these particular potential problems (see below).
- *Problem*: having to give each peer a different grade or mark.
- *Solution*: prior to the start of the placement, preparing students to accept that it is unlikely that they will both have exactly the same profile of skills can help in this eventuality (see below).
- *Problem*: not being able to differentiate between students.
- *Solution*: although feedback from the clinical teacher participating in the first pilot study suggested that this may be a problem, subsequent experience indicates that when two students are difficult to differentiate they in fact have very similar profiles of ability. Ensuring adequate opportunities to observe each peer working and some individual feedback/discussion time will facilitate differentiation of student profiles.
- *Problem*: an expectation that taking two students must create twice as much work.
- *Solution*: there is more work involved in planning a peer placement than planning a singleton placement (see below) and there is more work at the end, in that the clinical teacher has to complete two assessment forms rather than one. Clinician feedback indicates that during the actual placement, however, a peer placement feels like less work than a singleton placement.

- *Problem*: there could be a greater demand on the clinical teacher if both students are clinically weak.
- *Solution*: although logic suggests that having two weak students will be more work than one weak student, experience has shown this not to be the case. A student on a singleton placement who becomes aware that he or she is not meeting the required standards can quickly lose confidence and start to panic. Once this happens it becomes increasingly hard work for the clinical teacher to 'draw out' the student to establish what is known, in order to help the student build knowledge and skills. Two weak students can at least take comfort in the fact that they are not the only one! There will be less of an element of inadequacy and panic and so greater opportunity for the clinical teacher to build on what *is* known. Two weak students can be set tasks to work on together and can help each other to develop.

What is essential to ensure success of a peer placement?

One essential factor to ensure that a peer placement does indeed provide an effective and satisfying learning and teaching experience is thorough preparation. The first steps in preparation are to ensure that all parties have an understanding of the aim of a peer placement, familiarity with the model and an appreciation of the many benefits of this mode of placement. From this understanding and appreciation is likely to come a willingness to engage in thorough preparation and to approach any difficulties creatively.

The next step is to prepare students for the peer placement experience. As indicated in the section on problems and solutions above, many potential problems can be avoided through ensuring that students have anticipated them. A two-hour session that introduces students to the aim and model of a peer placement, outlines the benefits and identifies potential problems, is likely to suffice. It is helpful if students have identified their peers prior to the session so that potential problems can be discussed in peer pairs in the session. Any apparently insurmountable difficulties can then be discussed with the tutor (see Figure 3.2 for supporting handout).

Feedback from clinical teachers suggests that a similar induction to peer placements is beneficial to them. In addition, they have also found it helpful to have a clear indication of the planning necessary prior to the start of the placement (see Figure 3.3 for supporting handout). If clear written information is provided, however, clinical teachers can, of course, induct one another.

Another factor essential to the success of peer placements is flexibility. Once students and clinical teachers have an understanding of the

Peer placements – notes for students

Why have peer placements?

Two heads are frequently better than one! Discussing your observations and ideas with a peer who is sharing your experiences can be very beneficial to your learning. Having the support of a colleague who is at a similar stage in their learning can be very reassuring. Working with a colleague on a peer placement gives you natural opportunities to develop team-working skills.

Working together

Peer discussion

In the early stages of your training, peer discussion will focus on sharing observations and discussing clients [caveat: CONFIDENTIALITY]. You can also role-play taking case history information or practise administration of assessments with your peer. As you acquire theoretical knowledge you can help each other to link theory with practice and later on you will be able to plan therapy activities and/or sessions together.

Peer feedback

When you have gained some experience and are starting to develop ideas regarding therapeutic approaches or techniques, you will observe your peer working and be able to give him or her feedback and/or suggestions regarding the session. Prior to this stage, you can help your peer by making observations for him or her, recording assessment results, transcribing speech/language, keeping an eye on the timing of a session, for example.

It is always a good idea when giving feedback to your peer to ask what they thought of the session first. This will avoid potential friction caused by you telling them things they know perfectly well for themselves!

How to choose a peer

On weekly placements you are likely to choose your closest friend on the course and this may well work out fine. On block placements, however, it is probably better to go with someone whom you like and respect but not your best friend – it could be the end of a beautiful friendship! (see Cautions below). A peer placement is unlikely to work out well if you pair up with someone you dislike or feel intimidated by.

continues over

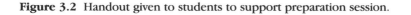

Figure 3.2 Handout given to students to support preparation session.

Cautions

Weekly placements

Time for peer discussion

As you may not be sharing accommodation with your peer (as in the case of block placements), you may not have the same opportunities to have your peer discussions. Your clinical teacher will organize time for these within the clinic session and university staff will ask you to sit with your peer for lecture or seminar discussion. You will also have opportunities to discuss your experiences with your peer in clinical tutorials. However, you will need time additional to these opportunities to have peer discussion and you must ensure that you organize time for this *each week*.

Block placements

Getting on

On a block placement you are likely to be sharing accommodation with your peer, and this has potential for problems. *Anticipate* that if you are spending 24 hours a day with someone, however much you like them, you are *likely* to get on each other's nerves at some point! Each of you may have different needs for personal space, so think about this *before* you go on the placement. Be aware of your own needs and consider how you can best prevent the build up of tension or how you will deal with it if it arises. Discuss this with your peer *before* the placement starts.

Any peer placement – weekly or block

Assessment

Accept before you commence your peer placement that you and your peer will have different skills and abilities. This means that you are likely to get different feedback from your clinical teacher and/or university tutor and you may get different marks at the end of the placement. Consider that if you were on a singleton placement you would not necessarily expect to get the same mark as your peer, so there is no reason why you should just because it is a peer placement. Having accepted that possibility, you need to consider how you will deal with the situation if you do get a different grade to your peer. It can be equally hard if your grade is higher or lower than your peer's, but anticipation of the possibility and consideration of how you will deal with it can make a significant difference to how you feel in this event. Again, discuss this possibility with your peer before you start the placement.

Getting enough attention

Some students have reported that they found themselves competing for their clinical teacher's time and attention on a peer placement. Try to remember that you are not in competition with one another, you are both there to learn and to develop and practise skills. If you begin to feel that your peer is receiving more time and/or attention than you, address the issue directly with your peer and, if appropriate, discuss it with your clinical teacher.

Figure 3.2 Handout given to students to support preparation session.

Planning for a peer placement

Peer placements can provide a more satisfying teaching experience for clinical teachers and a more satisfactory learning experience for students. Feedback from clinical teachers who have undertaken peer placements indicates that careful planning, prior to the start of the peer placement, is crucial to its success. Below are some guidelines, derived from experience to date, to aid in your planning. We would welcome feedback, which will contribute to the further development of these guidelines.

Plan time for:

- students to observe you working – all through the placement
- students to reflect on their observations
- students to have peer feedback and discussion
- you to listen to students' feedback and enhance discussion
- you to observe students working with clients
- you to feed back to students as peers *and individually*
- students to show you their session plans, ask questions, report back on tasks you have requested they undertake, etc. (half an hour at the beginning of each session (half-day) is ideal).

Figure 3.3 Handout for clinical teachers to support preparation session.

suggested model of peer placements and an appreciation that the aim is to facilitate students' learning, then confidence will develop to take a flexible approach to the model. Through creative adaptation of the original model, peer placements have operated successfully in schools, hospitals, child development centres, elderly residences, nurseries, day centres and many other clinical settings where clinicians work with groups of clients or where intervention is indirect.

Development of peer placements – peer-tutoring placements

The consensus opinion of clinical placement providers consulted in 1994 was that the best placement experience for students was a combination of weekly and block placements. In 1995, the speech and language therapy course at De Montfort University was reviewed and the structure changed to accommodate both types of placement. At the same time, all second-year weekly placements were organized into peer placements. In 1998, when the first cohort of students on the new course reached fourth year, the second-year first placement experience was changed into a peer-tutoring placement. Instead of second-year students being peer-placed with each other, each second year student was peer-placed with a fourth-year student.

Aims of peer-tutoring placements

Griffiths et al. (1995) undertook a pilot project to evaluate peer tutoring in a range of undergraduate modules. They reported that 96% of the students surveyed said that the peer-tutoring experience was enjoyable and worthwhile. Students identified that of particular benefit to them was the development of a complete range of personal transferable skills. The researchers also stated that there was substantial evidence that students had gained specific knowledge in their subject through peer tutoring. Fry et al. (2000) reported on academic peer support between first- and second-year undergraduates. They reported that the less experienced students benefit from an increase in confidence and self-esteem, resulting in improved study and cognitive skills. For the more experienced students they reported development of a range of skills, including transferable team leadership and communication skills, and deeper understanding of their own subject area. These benefits were anticipated to apply equally well to clinical placement peer-tutoring experiences.

For second-year students, the aim of peer-tutoring placements is the same as that for peer placements – to facilitate their learning. For fourth-year students the aim is to facilitate their transition from student to practising clinician by developing their confidence in their own knowledge and skills. When a student can pass on his or her knowledge, or teach another student to do something, he or she can be sure that he or she has that knowledge or skill himself or herself.

How do peer-tutoring placements work?

The aims and objectives for the second-year student are not changed because the fourth-year student is peered with them. The broad view of the roles of each participant in this placement is as follows:

- *Fourth-year student* supervises the second-year student on the placement. In large part, the fourth-year student adopts the previous role of the clinical teacher for the second-year student. For example, he or she helps them to identify areas for observation and discusses observations with them; demonstrates and discusses case-history taking, and informal and formal assessment; observes the student and provides feedback; discusses his or her own treatment with the second-year student; provides general support for the second-year student.
- *Second-year student*: the role for the second-year student remains as it was. The aims and objectives for second-year students are clearly stated and the second-year student fulfils these while on placement. The only difference for the second-year student is that they are peered with a fourth-year student who has more experience than they do themselves, rather than being peered with another second-year student.
- *Clinical teacher*: the clinical teacher supervises the fourth-year student's supervision of the second-year student, making sure that the fourth-year student knows what is expected of him or her and is confident to undertake the required tasks. The clinical teacher, of course, retains responsibility for both students, and observes both students working as well as observing the peer feedback sessions. It is the clinical teacher's role to complete each student's assessment form, but this may be done after consultation with each student regarding the other. For example, the clinical teacher may want to discuss with the fourth-year student the second-year student's skills in observation before completing that part of the assessment form.

(See Appendix 3.1 for a summary overview of the ten-week peer-tutoring placement.)

In addition to the teaching and support role while actually in the clinic setting, fourth-year students induct the second-year students into the placement prior to the start of it. They also plan and implement five one-hour tutorials, outside clinic time, for the second-year student. Fourth-year students are required to write a peer-tutoring report that outlines the plans and outcomes of these tutorials and reflects on their experience of peer tutoring. Fourth-year students are inducted into peer tutoring prior to their first meeting with their second-year peers (see Appendix 3.2 for supporting handout).

Feedback on peer-tutoring placement experiences

Peer-tutoring placements have proved to be extremely popular with all parties. Clinical teachers are very impressed with the fourth years' ability to nurture and guide the second-year students. They repeatedly report their appreciation of the fourth-year student's role in the development of the second-year student and state that the whole placement experience is eased for them in peer-tutoring placements (see Figure 3.4).

'Peer-tutoring has been a useful experience for all concerned. It has meant that we have all been reflective in our approach to treatment. It has given the fourth-year student confidence as she demonstrated knowledge to the second-year student. Also, the second-year student accepted advice more openly from the fourth-year student.'

'The peer-tutoring placement has been most successful with the students I've had. All three of us have found it enjoyable and have learned a great deal. Occasionally there have been difficulties juggling the different requirements of each student when there have not been sufficient or appropriate ward patients. I've found the peer process makes my feedback easier knowing that tutorials will take place between visits. The fourth-year student has supported the second-year well.'

'I felt the format is good, it enabled the fourth-year student to clarify ideas when giving feedback to the peer. It enabled both students to discuss aims and objectives together and think things through rather than having to make decisions alone. It helped take the pressure off me as it was much less formal than a student–clinician relationship, it became a joint effort.'

'I feel that the peer placement mix worked well, it provided useful experiences for both the second-year and final-year student. I also found it helpful to have the support of the final-year student as an aid to the second-year student.'

'Peer-tutoring enabled the 3+ student to use her knowledge of the course and material already covered to explain to the second-year student any information she didn't already have. The tutorials between the fourth-years and second-years seemed to work well.'

Figure 3.4 Examples of feedback from clinical teachers on their peer-tutoring experiences.

The second-year students find the support of their fourth-year peers invaluable. They unanimously express that they feel inspired through working with their fourth-year student and encouraged to know that they will be able to do that in 18 months' time (see Figure 3.5).

Fourth-year reflection indicates that most students feel some anticipatory anxiety prior to the induction meeting with their second-year peers. This anxiety is quickly dispelled in the meeting however, when the fourth-years realize the level of anxiety of the second-years and the nature of the questions that they ask. Fourth-years are reminded how little they knew

'I felt having a fourth-year peer was a VERY beneficial experience. Not only was it reassuring to know that any questions or queries could be answered and the extra help and support was there, it was also inspiring to think that 'one day' (maybe!) I too will be that knowledgeable and able to cope as well as my peer did with the challenges of clinic.'

'Very helpful to have a fourth-year peer. I don't think I would have had the experience I had if I had not had someone more experienced to help me. She was very helpful in reassuring me and explaining anything I wasn't sure about. She talked me through everything I had to do so I felt confident about it. I don't think I would have been so calm or gained so much if I had had to go on my own. She also helped me with other things such as university work, e.g. neurology, and was very reassuring that there is a light at the end of the tunnel and the course can be done!'

'The peer-tutoring arrangement worked very well for me. My peer was extremely supportive, shared her knowledge and guided me thoughtfully and sensitively through all aspects of the placement and associated assignments/tasks. A very valuable experience which I look forward to in the fourth year myself.'

'Unfortunately I didn't have a peer-tutoring placement or a peer placement and I feel that I would have felt more comfortable in clinic if that had not been the case. Although my clinical teacher was excellent and very approachable, I found it difficult to ask her questions. I realize this was no one's fault and understand that it could not be helped.'

Figure 3.5 Examples of feedback from second-year students on their peer-tutoring experience.

as second-years and how anxious they were before their first placement experience. They consistently report that the peer-tutoring experience does indeed facilitate the development of their confidence in their knowledge and skills. An added bonus reported by some students is that helping the second-year to fulfil the learning outcomes for their placement causes them to revisit aspects of their own work that they would not otherwise have done and affirm for themselves how much they know (see Figure 3.6).

Many fourth-years write in their reflective piece that having experienced a peer-tutoring placement they look forward to taking students on placement when they are practising clinicians. Feedback from second-year students, clinical teachers and university tutors suggests that they will be very competent to do so. Another way forward to solving the shortage of clinical placements?

'Overall peer tutoring was very beneficial – learned lots and realized how much I knew!'

'Overall the whole peer-tutoring experience was good. The experience taught me a lot about personal and clinical practice, encouraging team-work and development of new skills as well as the development of rapport. To summarize, the whole experience was fun for all of us and if given the opportunity I would happily repeat it.'

'I felt this was a very good experience for both of us. I enjoyed sharing my knowledge and it helped me to realize how much I knew.'

'It was a really useful experience and, although at times I did wonder if I was being of much help to my peer, I feel I have learned a lot and helped her too. I think it will be of real benefit when I come to have a student myself.'

'Having a peer on placement was a good experience for both of us. It made me realize my knowledge level and grow in confidence. It gave me the opportunity to practise explanations at an appropriate level for someone with very little knowledge. It was nice to see how my peer developed over the placement.'

'The most important thing about the peer-tutoring placement is that the students and clinician worked as a triangle not as a hierarchy. I think this was confidence building for both of us as we both felt we had equal attention from the clinician.'

Figure 3.6 Examples of feedback from fourth-year students on their peer-tutoring experience.

Acknowledgements

I would like to acknowledge the work of Jeannie Astill, who introduced and successfully implemented peer-tutoring with first- and third-year students during their university playgroup experience. Her work provided the inspiration and impetus for developing peer-tutoring clinical placements. Thanks to Pippa Noble for useful comments and eagle-eyed editing of the first draft of this chapter. I am also grateful for the careful editing advice received from Shelagh Brumfitt.

References

Best D, Rose M (1996) Quality Supervision: Theory and Practice for Clinical Supervisors. London: WB Saunders.

Fry H, Ketteridge S, Marshall S (2000) Handbook for Teaching and Learning in Higher Education. London: Kogan Page.

Griffiths S, Houston K, Lazenbatt A (1995) Peer Tutoring: Enhancing Student Learning through Peer Tutoring in Higher Education. Northern Ireland: University of Ulster.

Grundy K (1994) Peer placements: it's easier with two. CSLT Bulletin. 510: 10-11.

Kolb DA (1984) Experiential Learning: Experience as the Source of Learning and Development. London: Prentice Hall.

Ladyshewsky R, Barie S (1996) Measuring quality and cost of clinical education. Paper presented at the annual conference of the Higher Education Research Development Society of Australia, Perth, July.

Ladyshewsky R, Healey E (1990) The 2:1 Teaching Model in Clinical Education: A Manual for Clinical Instructors. Toronto: University of Toronto, Department of Rehabilitation Medicine

Lincoln M, Stockhausen L, Maloney D (1996) Learning processes in clinical education. In McAllister L, Lincoln M, McLeod S, Maloney D (eds) Facilitating Learning in Clinical Settings. London: Nelson Thornes.

McAllister L (1996) An adult learning framework for clinical education. In McAllister L, Lincoln M, McLeod S, Maloney D (eds) Facilitating Learning in Clinical Settings. London: Nelson Thornes.

Schon D (1987) Educating the Reflective Practitioner. San Francisco: Jossey-Bass.

Appendix 3.1
Level 3+ weekly peer-tutoring placement (W3) – an overview

Week	Level 2 student	Level 3+ student	Clinical teacher
0	Make contact with 3+S and CT	Make contact with 2S and CT	Students and UCT will contact you
1	*Observe CT with two clients* *Observe 3+S with one client* Discuss observations with 3+S	*Observe CT with two clients* *Discuss observations with 2S* Identify observation areas for 2S for next week Plan treatment for one client for next week	**Demonstrate treatment or informal assessment with two clients, one of which 3+S will take over treatment of next week** After students have had opportunity to discuss observations: – check 3+S has appropriate ideas for therapy – check 2S has appropriate observation areas
2	*Observe CT with one client* *Observe 3+S with one client* Discuss observations with 3+S	*Observe CT with one client* *Treat one client* Discuss 2S's observations and identify observation areas for next week Plan treatment for client for next week	**Demonstrate treatment or informal assessment with one client for 2S and 3+S to observe** After students have had chance to discuss, check 2S's observations and 3+S's session evaluation
3	*Observe CT with one client* *Observe 3+S with one client* Discuss observations with 3+S	*Observe CT with one client* *Treat one client* Discuss 2S's observations and identify observation areas for next week Plan treatment for client for next week	**Demonstrate treatment or informal assessment with one client for 2S and 3+S to observe** After students have had chance to discuss, check 2S's observations and 3+S's session evaluation Ensure 3+S is prepared for informal assessment *UCT will make telephone contact*

Code: CT = clinical teacher; UCT = university clinical tutor; 3+S = fourth-year student; 2S = second-year student

Bold type represents session with a client; *bold italic type represents observation sessions.*

Week	Level 2 student	Level 3+ student	Clinical teacher
4	*Observe 3+S with two clients* Present to CT observations on one client	**Treat one client** **Demonstrate informal assessment with one client** Discuss with 2S and ensure 2S is prepared for informal assessment next week	*Observe 3+S treating client* After students have had opportunities to discuss: – 2S presents observations on one client – 3+S feeds back outcome of informal assessment and progress of treatment of own client Complete appropriate sections of assessment forms and discuss with students
5	**Conduct informal assessment** *Observe 3+S with client* Discuss with 3+S	*Observe 2S* **Treat one client** Discuss with 2S	Listen to peer feedback, guiding students as appropriate
6	**Conduct informal assessment** Discuss with CT *Observe 3+S doing formal assessment* Discuss with 3+S	**Treat one client** **Demonstrate formal assessment with one client** Discuss with 2S; ensure 2S is prepared for formal assessment next week	*Observe 2S doing informal assessment*, give feedback and complete appropriate part of assessment form in discussion with students *Observe 3+S treating client*
7	**Conduct formal assessment** *Observe 3+S* Discuss with 3+S	**Treat one client** *Observe 2S conducting formal assessment* Discuss with 2S	Listen to peer feedback, guiding students as appropriate *UCT will make telephone contact*

Week	Level 2 student	Level 3+ student	Clinical teacher
8	**Conduct formal assessment** *Observe CT* Discuss with CT	**Treat one client** *Observe CT* Discuss with CT	**Demonstrate case-history taking** and discuss with students *Observe 2S* Give feedback and complete appropriate section on assessment form in discussion with students
9	**Conduct case-history taking** *Observe 3+S doing case history* Discuss with CT	**Conduct case history taking** *Observe 2S* Treat one client	*Observe 3+S and 2S doing case histories* Discuss with students
10	**Conduct case-history taking** *Observe 3+S treating client* Discuss with 3+S	**Treat one client** *Observe 2S* Discuss with 2S	*Observe 3+S treating client* *Observe 2S taking case history* Observe feedback session Complete assessment forms and give to students to return to the university

Appendix 3.2
Level 3+ professional development – handy hints for peer tutoring

Observation

Your peer will require quite specific guidance when observing in clinic. If asked simply to 'observe a session' he or she will not know what to note down and comment upon. You will recall that there is a list of functions, which may be observed and commented on, in the level 2, semester 1 placement information. Your role is to identify two or (maximally) three of these areas for your peer to focus on any time he or she is asked to observe. (You may wish to confer with your clinical teacher to decide appropriate areas.) For example, you might ask your peer to focus on a child's gross and fine motor skills and their concentration span; or you might ask him or her to focus on an adult's non-verbal communication and self-esteem.

When your peer has had a chance to organize his or her notes, it is important that he or she has the opportunity to feed back his or her observations to you and/or your clinical teacher. In the early stages of the placement we would anticipate that this feedback will be, broadly, a list of general observations marshalled under the specific headings agreed. Your role here is to teach your peer the significance of the observations he or she has made. Towards the end of the placement, therefore, we would expect your peer to be beginning to interpret his or her observations.

Caveats

It is very easy when asking a student for feedback to ask if he or she also noticed X or Y – perhaps something particularly interesting that you had just noticed yourself. If X or Y are not in the areas which you focused your peer to look at, it is unlikely that he or she *will* have noticed and he or she may well feel crestfallen. So, **Handy hint no. 1**: only probe your peer for detail in the areas defined prior to the session. If there was something you considered to be blatantly pertinent outside of the defined areas, give appropriate feedback on your peer's own observations and then use a general question such as '*Was there anything else of interest that you noticed?*'

You may find that your peer has made pertinent observations that passed you by. This can be unnerving, since you would generally expect to know more than your peer! **Handy hint no. 2**: it is helpful to remember that all your peer had to do in that session was to observe a small and specifically defined area of functioning while you, on the other hand.... Anticipate that he or she will notice things that you don't and, if it seems appropriate, let him or her know when this is the case and give praise.

Informal assessment

You will recall that your peer is required to conduct one receptive and one expressive informal language assessment. Your clinical teacher will have identified a client for whom these assessments will be beneficial and may well indicate a specific area for assessment and some broad suggestions for suitable types of activity. Your role will be to support your peer in his or her collation of informal assessment materials and assessment design. This may well be an appropriate area for one of your tutorials.

The purpose of this task is for your peer to learn about informal assessment and, although it may be tempting, it will not help his or her learning if you hand over your own informal assessments or design the assessment yourself. **Handy hint no. 3**: give your peer examples of informal assessments on areas that he or she is *not* being asked to assess and then get him or her to generate ideas for the areas that he or she is going to assess. You can then advise on the appropriacy of the suggestions. For example, if he or she is going to evaluate an individual's comprehension of verbs you could demonstrate a method of evaluating comprehension of nouns. **Handy hint no. 4**: we learn by our mistakes! It is not necessary for your peer's first attempt at informal assessment to be perfect. If you anticipate that one aspect of the assessment is unlikely to work, do not necessarily change it; your peer will learn more through working out for himself or herself how to improve it after conducting the assessment.

Formal assessment

As your peer is required to conduct one formal receptive language assessment and one formal expressive language assessment, this could be another topic for tutorial. You could ask your peer to familiarize himself or herself with a formal assessment and then role-play the assessment, with you as the client, in the tutorial.

Case-history taking

You and your peer should get the opportunity to observe your clinical teacher conducting a case-history interview. It will be helpful to your peer to discuss your observations together. Again, this may be an appropriate topic for a tutorial, and giving your peer the opportunity to role-play case-history taking with you may well increase his or her confidence for the actual task.

Feedback

After you have observed your peer undertaking the above tasks he or she will expect you to provide feedback. He or she will benefit from clear and direct feedback which is sensitively delivered – remember your assertiveness sessions in level 2 on giving and receiving criticism!

Handy hint no. 5: always take notes when observing your peer work. Give your peer some time to think about the task he or she has just undertaken before you start the feedback session. While he or she is thinking, organize your own notes. If you have several criticisms to make, try and identify two or three key points and ignore the rest – this will avoid overwhelming your peer, and the other points can be addressed at a later date. Try and ensure that you always have at least two positive points to make.

Handy hint no. 6: always ask your peer how he or she thinks the session went *before* you give your opinion – there is nothing worse than being told that you made an error when you know perfectly well for yourself that you did!

Handy hint no. 7: listen carefully to your peer's evaluation of the task and jot down notes rather than interrupting his or her flow if you want to discuss points with him or her.

Handy hint no. 8: you will probably find that your peer's evaluation is more negative than positive. It is very tempting to be reassuring and to deny all the negative views that your peer has. It will be more helpful to your peer if you lightly acknowledge where his or her evaluation is correct and then give reassurance. For example, you may say 'yes you did speak rather quickly, but you do well to be aware of it. I'm sure now that you are aware of it you will remember to speak a little slower next time.'

Handy hint no. 9: when it is your turn to give feedback you may offer your peer to have the good news or the bad news first ... not in those words of course! Although it may seem most appropriate to give the positive points first, it has been found through experience that some students prefer to have the negative points first as they do not listen to the positive because they are waiting for the negative. So, it may be helpful to say something like 'I have X things that I noticed that I thought were really good and Y things that I think you could develop – where would you like to start?'.

Handy hint no. 10: feel confident to give praise where you feel your peer has done something well and remember that where things have not been done so well, this is an opportunity for your peer to learn.

I hope you will find the above helpful in your peer-tutoring endeavours. Please do let me have feedback on the usefulness of these suggestions and if you have any handy hints to add, please let me have them!

Enjoy yourselves, Kim

Chapter 4
The transition from speech and language therapy student to newly qualified professional

SHELAGH BRUMFITT AND KIRSTEN HOBEN

Introduction

By the time a speech and language therapy student achieves a qualification, he or she will have reached the required standards of competence in knowledge, skills and attitudes. The newly qualified therapist will be expected to take responsibility for the caseload, and to assess, intervene and manage the client group. This includes professional autonomy, demonstrating the ability to work effectively within a team and with other professionals. In addition, the new clinician will be expected to work in a variety of contexts, which are complex and change frequently. Thus, the therapist needs to have generic skills (McAllister et al., 1997) that enable him or her to function in a changing environment. Influences on change may be political decisions, new decisions about the delivery of a service and interpersonal factors, such as multiprofessional approaches to the client, which require adaptation to different types of team working.

In consequence, the transition from student to professional may only be the beginning of developing into a confident experienced clinician. As Bray et al. (1999: p. 201) say, 'your learning now begins'.

How that transition takes place and what factors affect the outcome of the process of moving from a student to a qualified professional is something that still needs more research in the speech and language therapy context. This chapter explores the literature and reports on a study that has examined the process from a variety of perspectives.

Professional transition

The process of becoming a professional has been referred to as 'professional socialization' (Ewan, 1988; White and Ewan, 1991). This describes the transition between being a student and becoming a practitioner and having the necessary competence to do this. This concept covers not only actual professional 'skill', but also the capacity to function successfully in the work context, being able to communicate with other professionals, deal with the administrative and organizational aspects of the professional role, and make a comfortable 'fit' into the job. In effect, it refers to the concept of 'fit for purpose' as defined by the Higher Education Quality Council/National Health Service Executive (1996). That is, does the professional fit the employer's requirements? Fitness for purpose describes the knowledge, skills, attitudes and attributes necessary for a specific job. However, as Ilot and Murphy (1999) point out, within that description there are core or key skills such as adaptability or flexibility which are increasingly important in the workplace. These skills are less easy to define and, of course, less easy to teach.

The education of a speech and language therapist

The speech and language therapy qualification is a three-year or four-year undergraduate degree or a two-year master's award. The qualifying course has to be registered with and accredited by the Royal College of Speech and Language Therapists and the Health Professions Council. The content of the course is directed by the Royal College as the professional body, and it provides the newly qualified speech and language therapist with the capacity to work with all client groups that cover the scope of practice in this profession. Importantly, the curriculum and professional standards should be strongly related to the job requirements.

During the past 20 years the knowledge base about communication impairment has continued to develop and expand so that the newly qualified therapist has to be able to use a very wide range of competencies in order to respond to the needs of this wide client group. There can be a great deal of variation between the approaches to working with the full spectrum of client groups. For example, working closely with voice clients requires a knowledge base around: diseases of the ear, nose and throat; classification of voice disorders; knowledge of and competence in intervention approaches, which may include specific vocal techniques and counselling. In addition, the therapist has to have an understanding of head and neck surgery, dysphagic problems associated with this and the ways in which communication might be facilitated following radical surgery.

In complete contrast, the therapist who works closely with children who have developmental language problems will require a theoretical knowledge base around language processing, language development, child development, evaluation of language impairment, intervention approaches in language impairment, literacy, the implications of language impairment on educational progress and parental counselling skills.

Although some of these competencies can be developed at a post-qualification stage, the new therapist is still expected to have a superordinate understanding of these areas and all the other client groups, and in principle be able to respond to any type of client who is referred. All speech and language therapists work independently and autonomously and the responsibility for the caseload lies with the individual therapist. We recognize that the development from dependent student to independent practitioner is a highly vulnerable stage in a long-term career in speech and language therapy.

A survey by the American Speech and Hearing Association (Rosenfield and Kocher, 1998) explored the perceptions of educators, practitioners and supervisors in terms of their understanding of the role of the speech and language pathologist. Participants were asked to state where they believed 53 clinical activities and 85 knowledge areas should be taught in the curriculum – either at pre-qualification level in the university setting or the clinical setting and/or the post-qualification work context setting. Although general agreement was found, an area of common concern related to the location of the clinical areas of teaching. The educators ($n = 160$) appeared to be satisfied with the placing of individual subject areas; 95% of clinical activities and 95% of the knowledge areas were reported as being learned in the appropriate place. However, practitioners ($n = 1013$), clinical supervisors ($n = 153$) and clinic directors ($n = 176$) perceived that many more clinical activities and knowledge areas should be covered at the university stage. There was a major recommendation for there to be better dialogue between these groups so that future improvements at pre-qualifying and post-qualification could be made.

Making the transition to professional practice: healthcare professions

Various professional groups have examined the ways in which the student makes a successful transition into the work context. Jones et al. (2001) examined the perceptions of medical house officers (graduating 3 months earlier) and to supervisors of pre-registration house officers. The graduates ($n = 256$; response rate 66%) and the supervisors ($n = 194$; response rate 76%) were sent questionnaires. The graduates were asked 'How well did the course prepare you for ...?' and were given a list of broad areas of competence. They were also asked for their comments on more specific skills. There was also space for for a fuller written comment. The supervisors also received a questionnaire with similar questions: 'Please rate the PRHOs on their competence in ...'.

Overall, the results from this study indicated that there were differences between the perceptions of the house officers and the supervisors in terms of how well prepared they were for the professional context. The key aspects brought out in the paper relate to the following (Jones et al., 2001: p. 2):

- 'Pre-registration house officers (PRHOs) felt much better prepared for the broad areas of competence, such as communication, than for specific skills such as suturing.'
- 'Supervisors differed from graduates in their perceptions of graduates' competence in understanding disease processes. Graduates rated themselves more favourably.'
- 'Awareness of legal and ethical issues and understanding the purpose and practice of audit peer review and appraisal have been identified as areas of competence where graduates felt less well prepared.'
- 'The undergraduate course appeared to have only partly met its objective of preparing graduates for the PRHO year, although there may be inappropriate expectations on the part of the respondents for the level of competence expected in a new graduate.' (p. 579)

The important aspect in relation to this study is its relevance to the speech and language therapy profession in terms of the relationship between the curriculum and the job. Some aspects were sufficiently well covered in the medical course. However, there was evidence that others, such as ethical issues and informatics, were not covered well. The authors comment, however, that the expectations of both groups may well have been higher than what it is reasonable for a student to achieve by the end of a degree and again this may have relevance for us.

In a well publicized study, Goodfellow and Claydon (2001) examined the experiences of 122 final-year medical students with reference to eight clinical skills that are normally required of junior doctors. These skills included:

- taking a sample of blood from a vein in an arm
- taking a sample of blood from the artery at the wrist to measure its oxygen level
- rectal examinations
- stitching wounds.

A substantial number had little or no experience in some core skill. Almost a third had never practised applying a urinary catheter and more than half had 'negligible' experience in electrocardiography (in spite of the fact that junior doctors in Sheffield hospitals were expected to do between three and ten catheterizations and electrocardiograms a month). Additionally, when the qualified junior doctors were questioned about their experience over the first year, most did not recall receiving further training in these selected core skills. From the results reported here it was clear that these house officers did practise these skills during the first year of work, but this was done with inadequate training and no monitoring of whether the correct technique was being applied. Smith and Poplett

(2002) also reported an assessment of knowledge of 188 trainee doctors at six hospitals. This demonstrated significant gaps in the doctors' knowledge of signs of acute illness and life-saving techniques.

Other evidence from the literature shows us that preparation for the workplace is often difficult to achieve. Ewens et al. (2001) examined the experiences of newly qualified community nurses, one year on in practice. Although the nurses reported positive views about their roles, the study demonstrated that the nurses felt inadequately prepared for the work context, the pressures and the pace in the health service.

In a survey on the experiences of newly qualified social workers and supervisors totalling 700 students and 60 supervisors (Marsh and Triseliotis, 1996), about three-quarters of all newly qualified staff described themselves as ready for practice, but half suggested that work was different from their expectations. In addition, around half indicated that they had not felt well prepared for work by their course. Only 53% believed that their courses were well taught, with identified gaps in knowledge in certain areas, such as law, psychology and information technology. The survey also showed that too few staff were provided with support and training in their first year of work. Although the newly qualified staff received some induction, it was rarely perceived as relevant to their individual needs. If supervision was provided, over half of the respondents rated it as good, although there were differences in the views about the regularity of the supervision, the newly qualified staff believing it to take place far less frequently than the supervisors did.

Williams et al. (2001) examined the more specific area of the doctor–patient relationship and the transition from undergraduate to the pre-registration 'reality'. This study looked at the views of 24 pre-registration house officers with reference to the doctor–patient relationship and compared it to their original undergraduate expectations. Some differences were reported, the first of which were internal, where the house officer had begun to change views about what constituted a good relationship and what the definition of a 'professional' relationship meant. Others views could be described as 'external', where they were influenced by the views of their senior colleagues. For example, where the house officer attempted to develop and maintain a good relationship with a patient, this was often reported as being perceived as working too slowly. The conclusion from this study was that in spite of receiving a strong education in developing good doctor–patient relationships while on the undergraduate degree, the hospital-based culture appeared to prevent that knowledge and skill being used to its full potential.

Jackson (2003) investigated senior managers' views on the overall competence of newly qualified therapeutic radiographers, recruiting responses from 62 managers. The areas of competence assessed ranged from skill with technical procedures (such as dose calculations) to professional skill (such as giving information and instructions to patients). The survey showed that three newly qualified staff gave cause for concern in some aspects of their work. Many of the newly qualified staff, however, demonstrated higher-level skills associated with independent critical thinking and adaptability. The therapeutic radiographer with a first class degree is, according to the results from the survey, likely to be a positive indicator for a high standard of performance.

Making the transition to professional practice: teachers

There is a large literature on the first year of work for the newly qualified teacher; a career phase which has been shown to affect job satisfaction, career length and teaching effectiveness (Hebert and Worthy, 2001). It is recognized that understanding this important first year can provide insights and outcomes relating to lifelong learning in the teaching context and also the overall quality of teacher education. Research in this area has focused on a series of perspectives.

First, socializing factors have been shown to be influential. These cover aspects such as the type of teacher education and the impact of the cultural 'norm' of the school, and how well the new teacher adjusts to that new environment. Also, more recently, the way in which the teacher engages with the school environment has been shown to be an influential factor. A second area of research has focused on the actual problems and difficulties experienced by teachers in their first post. Hebert and Worthy (2001) describe these as difficulties associated with managing student behaviour, time management and planning appropriate lessons. Additional problems described include the new teacher being expected to assume the same responsibilities as the more experienced teacher, being given a heavy workload, and being given little support and mentoring. Finally, how new teachers find a place for themselves in the political organization of a school has been reported as another aspect that can affect the success of the transition.

Hebert and Worthy describe five issues which provide explanations for the difficulties found in this first year of work.

- Unrealistic expectations and beliefs about teaching the children/students, the workplace and the difficulty of teaching in general.
- Limitations of teacher education programmes; this has been criticized for failing to educate students in the real-life aspects of the work with the children.
- Student teaching experiences, which are intended to link the higher education training with the workplace. These have been criticized for providing only a restricted experience for the student teacher; in that the student is shielded from the more difficult aspects of teaching, and experiences this without needing to be aware of the organizational structure of the school and avoids administrative responsibilities.

- Features in the school environment also appear to influence outcome; the beginning teacher may be given difficult class assignments with little support and be expected to function in a school which is 'unable or unwilling to provide nurture and support' (Deal and Chapman, 1989).
- The personal characteristics of the teacher which may impede their progress into professional life. These include poor interpersonal abilities with both children and colleagues. (p. 899)

In contrast to these areas of difficulty, there are clearly new teachers who do cope well with the first year and find it a positive experience. If no teacher did so, then the attrition rate would be impossible to manage. However, as Hebert and Worthy point out, there is comparatively little work done in this area.

Schmidt and Knowles (1995) discuss four cases of female novice teachers who perceived themselves as 'failures'. Although only one actually failed the student teaching component, all four subsequently chose alternative careers. Schmidt and Knowle's paper looks at the novice teachers' explanations for why they perceived themselves as failing. The methodological approach included participant observation and regular interviews with novice teachers, and each teacher keep a semi-structured journal recording reactions to her experiences.

Four main clusters of factors emerged from the qualitative analysis of all these data. First, 'personal histories' are reported as important influences in the teachers' overall perceptions. Although the teachers were described as coming from diverse backgrounds, all four reported poor or negative experiences in their own school education. All four recalled feeling shy and socially awkward and experienced the same feelings returning when they began their teaching experience.

Second, the experience of 'self as teacher' was found to have an impact. Three of the teachers had approached classroom teaching on the basis that teaching in class was similar to being a 'camp counsellor' where a 'buddy' relationship could develop. The fourth teacher had worked previously as a church missionary and reported having approached classroom teaching in the same way as she would have worked with small groups. Both of these strategies caused problems, and in spite of feedback from supervisors, all felt changing to 'being a teacher' was difficult.

Instructional and management concerns were also identified as problematic. In this category there was evidence for all four teachers finding it difficult to respond to instruction and advice from mentors and supervisors. Mentors reported that the teachers 'had not heard' the advice, were 'unwilling to learn' or had 'no desire to improve themselves', in spite of all the teachers stating they wanted to be told what to do.

Finally, the actual teaching context appeared to be influential. There was evidence that the teaching practice had been poorly matched with their perceived needs and goals. None of the four teachers was given a place in her major subject area, they had a heavy schedule which allowed little time for reflection or recreation, and the experience left them physically and emotionally weak. In addition, some of the mentors had poor skills. The authors of this paper concluded that further work is needed to explore the interactions between all of these identified factors.

The speech and language therapy context

In a recent study on the experiences of newly qualified speech and language therapists and the perceptions of their employers (Brumfitt et al., 2002), five key conclusions were drawn from the survey results. These conclusions were reached by three studies:

- in-depth interviewing of senior managers
- questionnaire survey to newly qualified speech and language therapists
- three focus groups created to follow up on the results from the first two studies, in order to triangulate the process.

Each of the conclusions will be considered below.

The role of core skills in the early stages of independent practice

Thirty-one newly qualified respondents completed the questionnaire, and nearly 70% reported that they were not confident with their skills on starting work. In terms of their specific difficulties in coping with the work context, 58% reported that organizing their day-to-day workload had proved extremely difficult. Additionally, the number of clients they were expected to deal with had proved to be a shock (38% of respondents). Other factors that newly qualified staff reported concerned the amount of sudden responsibility they were expected to take on, the experience of having to work in isolation and the lack of opportunities to plan their work in advance. This same group of newly qualified therapists also reported that their main concern on starting work had been their responsibility for effective client management – that is, would their therapeutic skills achieve the desired outcome?

All these questionnaire data are reflected in the focus group of newly qualified therapists who completed this part of the study. The type of comments that reflected their anxiety related to actual accuracy of intervention and to other work-related skills, such as administrative ability. The comments included:

- 'Your ultimate nightmare is to miss something really.'
- 'I mean in clinical placements, you get to see a few patients and that's about it; you don't get to do any sort of admin, you don't get to do the day-to-day running of a clinic or your own caseload, you don't get to do any sort of caseload management or prioritization.'

- 'Non-clinical skills are down to your personality and your own skills as well.'
- 'I mean, I think some of my administrative skills came from things I'd done before, you kind of pick things up from being in other environments don't you?'

Although the newly qualified in this group recognized the need to be organized and to be a fully independent professional, there were difficulties associated with their perceived skill base. Many of the comments reflected the view that they were relying on previous work experience (including summer jobs) to cope with the organizational demands of the job. These sorts of skills appeared to have been given limited time at the pre-qualification stage, although it was stated that there was some variation between qualifying courses. Additionally, the experience in prioritization and caseload management was enhanced if the student was given a placement with a supervising therapist who was able to spend time on this aspect.

The senior managers' focus group, which consisted of managers from outside the region used in the study, reported concerns about lack of preparation on the pre-qualifying courses in time management, organization and liaison within the work context. Students were seen as having few opportunities for real-life report writing and case note maintenance.

The managers from the original interviews also commented on the need for more generic workplace skills and reflected an awareness that this was often difficult to provide in the university setting.

Therapeutic intervention skills

In the interviews with 13 managers of speech and language therapy services (Brumfitt et al., 2002) a key concern related to the newly qualified therapists' clinical competence. A strong view was expressed that students needed a wide range of clinical experiences and clinical teaching before qualifying and working in independent practice. It was noted that there were some areas that were not covered as thoroughly as others at the pre-qualification level, such as learning disabilities.

These concerns have often been expressed in the speech and language therapy context. Comments about 'being too academic' are heard frequently. Qualifying courses in universities are often accused of focusing too strongly on the classification and fine description of speech and language therapy impairment while paying limited attention to the intervention process. Comments were also made around the universities' focus on developing research skills at the expense of developing practical skills. In the higher education field, there is often discussion about where the teaching of clinical skills should occur. For example, should it be before the theoretical teaching or afterwards? A further debate centres around the issue of whether it is even the universities' responsibility to teach this or whether it should be done externally by the clinicians. As the ASHA study (Rosenfield and Kocher, 1998) demonstrated, there is something of an unresolved dispute about whether the responsibility lies with the university at the pre-qualification stage or whether the development of clinical skills should only take place post-qualification. In the ASHA study, four groups were surveyed: educators, practitioners, clinical fellowship supervisors and clinic directors, totalling 1502 actual respondents to an extensive questionnaire. One part of the survey investigated views on the relevance of clinical activities and knowledge areas to the job. Strong agreement was found between the groups. However, when asked to state where the clinical activities and knowledge areas should be learned, there was much less agreement. Educators perceived that 95% of the clinical activities and 95% of the knowledge areas were being learnt in the appropriate place. The views of the other three groups focused on the need for more clinical activities being at the university stage.

Brumfitt et al.'s 2002 study found that the majority of managers reported that it was the universities' responsibility to develop further professional competence by teaching skills before the therapist arrived in the workplace, but recognized the difficulty of making this a reality:

> If we are going to have a training course which trains therapists to work in any kind of environment, then hoping that therapists are going to feel totally proficient in everything when they come out is probably not realistic. (managers' focus group)

This comment represents the noted tension between preparing the newly qualified speech and language therapist to face any aspect of professional work versus the practical impossibility of doing this. This theme was repeated throughout the interviews and focus groups with all managers.

In addition, during the interview process with managers, they were asked to state how they made the judgement about the newly qualified's clinical competence after starting work. Twenty-five percent of managers reported that they used the appraisal after the first six months of employment to make a judgement, but that they also took into account feedback from others (31%), peer review (31%) and case note audit (13%). The factors that the managers reported as creating an increase in clinical competence after starting work, were the level of support the therapist received (85%), the personal qualities of the therapist (46%) and their previous real-life experiences (46%). The difficulty of accommodating those factors into the pre-qualification course needs further debate, and may influence decisions at the selection stage.

When a focus group of newly qualified therapists discussed the issue of their therapeutic intervention skills there was a strong recognition of how unskilled they felt in their first few weeks at work, but that they found that these skills did develop over time. Specific examples were discussed in this group, such as the therapist who failed to notice and assess an aspect of the child's behaviour which was critical to the diagnosis. There was also the therapist who had to see a child in a classroom but found the teacher would not listen to advice or even acknowledge that the child had a special problem. Another therapist discussed the difficulty of arriving in a challenging post in learning disabilities having only done a one-week placement in that context before qualifying.

Support for the newly qualified in the work context

The newly qualified speech and language therapists reported a lack of adequate support in their work context owing to limited opportunities for peer support, made worse by a lack of a shared base. Also, infrastructure in the service to support supervision and mentoring of the newly qualified was rare. Of the 31 therapists who returned the questionnaire, only 23% reported that they received a monthly formalized supervision session. Twenty-three percent reported that they had received no formally organized supervision at all.

Sixty-eight percent of the therapists who returned the questionnaire reported peer support as being a critical factor in increasing professional competence after qualification. In a subsequent focus group, other newly qualified speech and language therapists reported the need for the increased responsibility on the part of the employer to create opportunities for supervision, peer support and mentoring, with time being allowed for this within the expectations of the daily workload. Comments about this need included:

- 'My experience of mentoring and supervision has been really good, but I've been the one that's had to ask for it.'
- 'I have a sort of mentor, she's there for me you know, but she's a kind of equal to me. Well I've met her once actually.'
- 'I think it depends on your set up. Because I was stuck in a clinic on my own, so that makes a difference because actually you're not meeting anybody else in the day.'

The experience of physical isolation by speech and language therapists was frequently referred to and is something other professional groups may not share. For example, as stated earlier, many speech and language therapists play a peripatetic role by visiting children and teaching staff in schools, or working in acute settings in hospitals. For the newly qualified therapist this can be extremely challenging. Comments from the focus groups highlight this special circumstance:

- 'It's because I feel a complete idiot going into the classroom, I just feel inferior to the teachers. In clinic I'm fine.'
- 'It's like working in a hospital, you're on a ward and it's like someone else's "territory".'

The influence of the past placement experience was also considered in relation to the need for support in the first post. Several members of the focus group believed that confidence gained in the clinical placement pre-qualification could affect how much support was needed in the first work context:

- 'I think if you've had positive, encouraging clinicians on your most recent clinical placements who've built you up and said, "you know with support you can do this", I think that gives you the encouragement to make that first step, if you've had really good placements.'

The need for support was recognized by the managers in the interview study (Brumfitt et al., 2002), with 85% reporting support as being a factor leading to an increase in clinical competence after starting work. The difficulty with this situation appears to be partly a resourcing issue; that is, is there 'free' time in the working week to provide opportunities for creating a supervision system for the newly qualified? Additionally, there is the issue of the culture in the profession. That is, many senior therapists had to develop their clinical competence and confidence without the benefit of supervision and mentoring and so see less need for this than the new therapists do.

The quality of clinical placements and supervisors

The project reported by Brumfitt et al. (2002) confirmed many of the beliefs about the importance of clinical placements and the increasing emphasis on quality assurance of placements. All respondents in this study stated their concern about, and belief in, the importance of the placement experience (groups of managers interviewed, newly qualified therapists questioned and focus groups). Eighty-five percent of the interview group of managers stated their belief that block placements were the preferred approach to clinical learning. Eighty-one percent of the newly qualified group rated their clinical placements as being critical in their capacity to cope in the first post. When asked to state their most useful clinical learning experiences, 61% of the newly qualified therapists stated that being observed while implementing a session was most important. The process of clinical supervision and feedback was rated by 51% as being very important.

In the following focus group with newly qualified therapists, again support for the block placement experience was expressed. The success of the placement experience appeared to be related to the personal experience of the student in working with the clinical teacher or supervising therapist. Some new therapists reported difficult experiences which had subsequently influenced the way they felt about themselves:

- 'For my last two placements I had really different clinicians, one of whom was like just not supportive at all and one who was really supportive and you know, if I'd had them the other way round then I'd be a wreck now but luckily I had them the better way round.'

- 'One of the reasons I don't want to work with [client group X] is because I had a really bad clinician in one of my placements and she knocked all the confidence out of me when working with [client group X]'.
- 'I got an absolute torrent of abuse throughout the ten weeks.'
- 'She wasn't like, "oh you should be knowing that by now"; she was like you know, "I've done it too". It made me feel like ... great, it didn't make me feel pushed out.'
- 'I think that universities have a responsibility to make sure that the placements we get are positive learning experiences, not confidence-knocking experiences.'

From the above quotations it can be seen that there are some strong views on the quality of clinical placements and the responsibilities associated with providing these placements. Senior managers from outside the region who formed a focus group, recognized the great importance of the clinical placement but expressed concern that it represented the 'real' working context. One factor that appeared to have influenced the experience for students related to NHS governance on 'risk' and how much (or how little) responsibility could be given to someone of student status. This was perceived as limiting the pre-qualification experience. This focus group suggested that the last six months of a qualifying degree should be devoted to placement-only experience, or if this could not be provided, then an intern year post-qualification should be mandatory.

Access to speech and language therapy qualifying courses

This project identified concerns about the narrow entry into the professional courses. Increasingly, speech and language therapy students had been selected because of strong academic profiles. There were several reasons for this. The courses were of an academically high standard and it was important to select students who had the intellectual ability to deal with this. Several of the courses were postgraduate and selected candidates on the basis of a good first degree, because the courses were two years in length and students required high-level learning skills to cope with the intensity of the learning experience. The project found that managers were particularly concerned that the entry routes for mature candidates, those from ethnic minority groups and those with non-standard academic backgrounds were extremely limited. A strong recommendation was for therapists at managerial level to be involved in the selection process of candidates.

Concern was expressed in the managers' focus groups about the need for appropriate social skills, given that some newly qualified therapists were viewed as being 'poor' with people.

It's all very well to say you choose someone that likes being with people, but you also need to choose someone that people like being with. (managers' focus group)

Comments were also made about the need for selecting people with 'common sense', such as having the ability to apply the academic material to the practical situation and not (example given from group) of going to a home visit where a child is being sick and demanding to do an assessment.

Additional concerns were expressed about the route for qualifying and the impact this had on speech and language therapy assistants who had proved themselves to be very able. Part-time routes were discussed, but there was some concern about the length of time needed to qualify on a part-time route (which could be as much as seven years). A suggestion was made for developing a modular route so that speech and language therapy assistants could gain some specialist qualifications to work in their particular context without needing to obtain the whole qualification.

Conclusions

All the research referred to here, in all the different professions, confirms the fact that the process of becoming a competent and comfortable professional takes time. Learning to use technical skill, whether it be taking blood, organizing a room of children for a whole day or diagnosing a developmental communication problem, takes up a huge amount of the student's and then the newly qualified therapist's attention. This has to be married with the development of sound interpersonal skills, which are context specific; a knowledge of the professional service; and a capacity to deal with the unexpected. There is plenty of evidence in the literature to show that newly qualified therapists have emerging skills which need time and a safe work experience to develop more fully. Their development may be based on a 'pure' academic ability – that is, those with the highest IQs do best in the long term. Or it may be based on a range of other factors:

- Personal factors, which are not about IQ but about attitude to learning.
- Factors related to the higher education experience, whether the student has a good or bad set of learning experiences.
- The context in which the newly qualified therapist first takes up a post. This may be critical to the future outcome.

What is important for our future understanding is to find a way of identifying 'markers' which would allow us to recognize when a newly qualified therapist is 'vulnerable'. Although we may recognize this through experience, it still needs establishing more rigorously through research.

As Ewan (1988) suggests, professional socialization develops through the interactions students have with colleagues, which become more focused over time and enable them to have a fuller understanding of what is required. This process appears to continue into post-qualification working life, but we need further evidence to identify the critical factors in this process. This has been identified by Lincoln and McAllister (1993) and also by Grundy; that peer learning may enable students to develop professional identity and may contribute to that developing understanding of how to function as a professional in the workplace.

To conclude, professional transition and successful socialization are complex and multifaceted. Brumfitt et al. (2002) found that only 29% of the newly qualified speech and language therapists in their survey believed they had fully understood the nature of what 'being a therapist' meant. Nearly 40% believed it was an ongoing process.

References

Bray M, Ross A, Tod, C (1999) Speech and Language Clinical Process and Practice. London: Whurr.

Brumfitt SM, Hoben K, Enderby P, Goddard V (2002) Informing educational change to improve the clinical competence of speech and language therapists. Final report. University of Sheffield.

Deal TE, Chapman RM (1989) Learning the ropes alone: socialising the new teachers. Action in Teacher Education 11: 21–29.

Ewan CE (1988) The social context of medical education. In Cox K, Ewan CE (eds) The Medical Teacher, 2nd edn. Edinburgh: Churchill Livingstone, pp. 85–89.

Ewens A, Howkins E, McClure L (2001) Fit for purpose: does specialist community nurse education prepare nurses for practice? Nurse Education Today 21: 127–135.

Goodfellow PB, Claydon P (2001) Students sitting medical finals – ready to be house officers? Journal of the Royal Society of Medicine 24: 516–520.

Hebert E, Worthy T (2001) Does the first year of teaching have to be a bad one? A case study of success. Teaching and Teacher Education 17: 897–911.

Higher Education Quality Council/National Health Service Executive (1996) Improving the Effectiveness of Quality Assurance Systems in Non Medical Health Care Education and Training. London: HEQC.

Ilot I, Murphy R (1999) Success and Failure in Professional Education: Assessing the Evidence. London: Whurr.

Jackson C (2003) Undergraduate learning in therapeutic radiography: a curriculum model for clinical education. Unpublished thesis, University of Derby.

Jones A, McArdle PJ, O'Neill PA (2001) How well prepared are graduates for the role of preregistration house officer? A comparison of the perceptions of new graduates and educational supervisors. Medical Education 5: 578–580.

Lincoln M, McAllister L (1993) Facilitating peer learning in clinical education. Medical Teacher 15: 17–25.

McAllister L, Lincoln M, McLeod S, Maloney D (1997) Facilitating Learning in Clinical Settings. Cheltenham: Stanley Thornes.

Marsh P, Triseliotis J (1996) Ready to Practise? Social Workers and Probation Officers; Their Training and Their First Year in Work. Aldershot: Avebury.

Rosenfield M, Kocher G (1998) The practice of speech-language pathology. A study of clinical activities and knowledge areas for the speech language pathologist. American Speech and Hearing Association website (www.Asha.org).

Schmidt M, Knowles JG (1995) Four women's stories of 'failure' as beginning teachers. Teaching and Teacher Education 11: 429–444.

Smith B, Poplett N (2002) Knowledge of aspects of acute care in trainee doctors. Postgraduate Medical Journal 78: 335–338.

White R, Ewan C (eds) (1991) Clinical Teaching in Nursing. London: Chapman and Hall.

Williams C, Cantillon P, Cochrane M (2001) The doctor–patient relationship: from undergraduate assumptions to pre-registration reality. Medical Education 35: 743–747.

PART II
SPECIFIC EDUCATIONAL CONTEXTS

Chapter 5
Approaches to teaching dysphagia to speech and language therapy students

SUE POWNALL

Introduction

Dysphagia is an abnormality of swallowing fluids or food. It can result from a wide range of neurological and structural disorders, for example after a head injury, in individuals with degenerative conditions such as motor neurone disease or Parkinson's disease, as a symptom of some cognitive disorders and in some psychiatric disorders. Dysphagia is reported to occur in approximately 45% of patients with stroke, and various studies also suggest that between 50 and 75% of nursing home residents have some difficulty with swallowing (O'Loughlin and Shanley, 1998). It is likely also that as the percentage of people over 70 years old increases, the incidence of dysphagia will increase accordingly as a symptom of advanced age. This will have direct implications for services providing care to older people. Dysphagia is a complex disorder that can lead to many other medical complications, including dehydration, malnutrition, airway obstruction, aspiration, life-threatening pneumonia and death. Sixty percent of deaths due to pneumonia are secondary to dysphagia-related aspiration (Kohler, 1991).

In addition to the medical factors, dysphagia impacts on a person's quality of life and psychological wellbeing. Social activities and routines may be disrupted, which can result in the person feeling increasingly isolated and socially excluded. The psychological impact also often spreads across the whole family as the dysphagia's effects extend beyond mealtimes and the dysphagic individual him- or herself. Often the spouse or carer's social activities, such as meals out with friends or a drink in the pub, are curtailed because of his or her partner's inability to join in the activity.

Over the past decade, speech and language therapy services have experienced a dramatic increase in the number and rate of dysphagic referrals and the field of dysphagia assessment and management is commonly thought to be the largest growth area for the speech and language therapy profession. Giles and Davison (1996) quoted an increase in referrals to the Newcastle General Hospital and Newcastle Royal Infirmary of 71% and 68% respectively in the preceding two years. This rate of increase has been mirrored for speech and language therapy departments on a national basis, and for many has continued on an upward trend since that time. This sharp increase in referrals appears to reflect the increase in awareness of and concern about the associated risks by medical and other healthcare professionals.

It is well recognized in the literature that early recognition of dysphagia can minimize or prevent complications including malnutrition, improve patient outcomes and reduce the cost of hospital care. Patients with aspiration pneumonia have been shown to stay in hospital on average 5.5 days longer than other patients, and the incidence of aspiration pneumonia due to dysphagia has been shown to be reduced from 6.7% to 0% through effective management (Odderson et al., 1995). Effective management depends on careful assessment of each patient's swallowing abilities and the presence of specific conditions or behaviours observed before, during and after feeding. Hence more and more pressure is being placed on speech and language therapy services to provide timely input to patients.

In November 1997, the Scottish Intercollegiate Guidelines Network produced a pilot edition of guidelines for the identification and management of dysphagia in stroke patients. They recommended that: 'All stroke patients should be screened before being given food or drink, to identify those patients with dysphagia.' Should any abnormalities of swallowing be identified then there should be an 'immediate referral to a speech and language therapist ... for a more detailed functional examination of swallowing'.

Most speech and language therapy services work to the standards set out by their professional body, the Royal College of Speech and Language Therapists (RCSLT), which states that 'In-patient referrals will be seen within two working days of receipt of referral, out-patient referrals within two weeks.' However, speech and language therapy services are finding these standards increasingly difficult to meet in many areas, even though most patients, carers and referrers would see this standard as too long already. In reality, two working days for inpatients may often mean a wait of four days over a weekend or longer over bank holiday periods.

This situation has already resulted in several cases being highlighted in the press. In 1997, Martin Bright, a journalist, wrote an article in the *Observer* entitled 'She was dying for a cuppa. Literally.' This article was about his grandmother, who had been admitted to hospital on a Friday night but was unable to have a drink until she had had her swallowing abilities assessed by a speech and language therapist. Unfortunately, the therapist was unable to carry out the assessment until the following week. This situation is partly, but not wholly, a consequence of speech therapists being funded to work only Monday to Friday 9am to 5pm. In 1998, the

Health Advisory Service in its document *Not Because They're Old*, recommended that swallowing assessments carried out by appropriately trained personnel should be available seven days a week.

Speech and language therapy involvement in dysphagia

The involvement of speech and language therapists in the assessment and management of patients presenting with dysphagia has a long history, and is often described as having developed from their work with children with physical and learning disabilities who have feeding difficulties. In 1990, a working party from the RCSLT produced a position paper, which aimed to clarify the role of speech and language therapists in the management of dysphagia and made recommendations regarding good clinical practice. Two years later, in 1992, the RCSLT held its first policy review forum in order to provide an arena in which to respond to issues affecting the profession. The topic of dysphagia was chosen as at that time concerns were already being raised by some members around the issue of the involvement of the profession with the treatment of dysphagia in people presenting with neurological disorders (O'Leary 1991; Dobinson and Parr, 1991).

At the forum a number of major concerns were expressed in relation to the rapid increase in dysphagia referrals and the escalating demand for dysphagia services. The concerns were published in the *College of Speech and Language Therapists Bulletin* in 1993 in an article by White et al. and included:

- Adequate training and experience of therapists carrying out dysphagia services.
- The role of speech and language therapists with this client group in relation to other healthcare professionals.

The article highlighted some of the views of the delegates at that time, including the idea that 'work with dysphagic patients enhanced professional status and provided a vehicle for improving services for all people with communication disorders'. It is often easier to demonstrate the successful endpoint in dysphagia management in a client with an acquired disorder than it is to show the same progress in a client with a communication disorder.

During the forum concerns were expressed about 'the level of competence expected of newly qualified therapists working in this area and the support they receive'. The question was also raised as to whether the position of making dysphagia a post-qualification training requirement was tenable. It was reported that 'grave concerns were expressed about the adequacy of the undergraduate curriculum on dysphagia and the difficulty in obtaining adequate practical experience during training'.

Recommendations made to the RCSLT following the forum included one for the College to 'consider urgently the level of undergraduate training in dysphagia and to promote the more rapid development of post-qualification courses and advanced courses in dysphagia'.

Until recently, the clinical area of dysphagia and the requirement to achieve dysphagia competencies have not been specific requirements of the pre-registration speech and language curriculum, resulting in a mismatch between the knowledge base and practical skill of new clinicians and what is now required of them in their working practice. Although some qualifying speech and language courses offered some dysphagia theory and hence gave the students a basic knowledge base, the content of these components varied widely. *Communicating Quality 2* (RCSLT, 1996) states that 'the speech and language therapist with specific responsibilities for dysphagia must have attended post-graduate education training at a post-basic level which includes consideration of:

- normal eating behaviour
- sensorimotor processes involved in self-feeding
- neurophysiological mechanisms of swallowing
- characteristic symptoms of the common causes of dysphagia and associated eating disorders.'

The post-qualification courses were required to be equivalent to at least one week's full-time tuition and to include a period of experiential learning, where clinical practice is supervised by an experienced colleague. Many therapists who had been qualified for many years felt that they had developed these dysphagia skills over time within their working practice and as such were expected to be able to demonstrate competence comparable to that provided by available courses. Over more recent years, the RCSLT has been registering short courses which enable participants to acquire these skills in a structured and supervised manner, and a small number of these courses have also become credit rated via universities in order to give participants credits towards a higher level or masters qualification.

This situation where postgraduate training is required to work within the specialism resulted in the question being raised by service managers as to whether newly qualified speech and language therapists were seen as 'fit-for-purpose'. If the majority of the workload within the adult patient service involves assessment and management of patients presenting with dysphagia, it is surely unacceptable that newly qualified therapists are unable to work within this clinical area. This situation also restricts the number of speech and language therapy vacancies that newly qualified therapists can apply for because many posts require the therapist to be trained in the field of dysphagia. Many departments which are already stretched to the limit in terms of maintaining their standards for seeing referrals often have little time or energy to support newly qualified therapists to a satisfactory level and thus need colleagues to be able to work independently with clients.

The professional requirement

In a response to this dilemma and to the issues raised by the Dysphagia Policy Review Forum (1999), the RCSLT Advanced Studies Committee produced a paper which made recommendations for pre- and post-registration dysphagia education and training. Their recommendation was that course providers introduce dysphagia into the curriculum as soon as possible, with the aim that students admitted for the academic year 1999–2000 would achieve the required competencies during their course. The committee felt that 'making the dysphagia content of pre-registration courses more explicit would enable newly qualified therapists to approach this clinical area with greater confidence'. Courses would be required to give students the necessary knowledge and skills to enable them to enter the profession with the basic competences to work within this clinical field under the supervision of an appropriately experienced practitioner. To achieve this recommendation it was expected that the curriculum would include the following knowledge base:

- anatomy and physiology of the head and neck
- neurology and neurophysiology, including the neurology of swallowing and the coordination of respiration, swallowing and phonation
- the normal swallow
- the aetiology of dysphagia
- key terms in dysphagia
- the referral process and case history
- associated legal issues and the ethics of decision making
- risk management, including health and safety
- awareness of the needs of clients with complex conditions, including tracheostomy, ventilator dependents and rare conditions.

Some of these areas would easily be incorporated into existing course components. For example, the anatomy and physiology of the head and neck is already included in many pre-registration curricula and is usually taught during the first year. The relevance and importance of this area could easily be flagged up as a pre-requisite for acquiring dysphagia competencies. Students often regard anatomy and physiology as dry and uninspiring. However, in relation to the teaching of the swallowing mechanism, the use of anatomical three-dimensional models can make these concepts become more meaningful. There are also excellent interactive CD-ROMs of the anatomy and physiology of normal swallowing available which can be used by individual students or small groups to aid learning and enhance the more traditional 'chalk-and-talk' style of learning.

Other aspects of the required knowledge base, such as the neurology of swallowing and the developmental influences on the swallowing mechanism across the life span, could also be incorporated into existing curricula without too many changes and again could be flagged up as prerequisite knowledge for working within the specialism.

Students would also be expected to have knowledge of the assessment and management of dysphagia including:

- oropharyngeal assessment, including manual assessment of the pharyngeal swallow
- commonly used assessments, which will include trial of food consistencies
- the role of instrumental assessment, e.g. videofluoroscopy, fibreoptic endoscopic examination of swallowing
- management strategies, including compensatory techniques, positioning and food consistencies
- service delivery, including multidisciplinary working and caseload management issues
- prognostic indicators
- consideration of environmental factors and the role of carers
- awareness of non-oral feeding options.

Depending on the structure of the pre-registration course, this knowledge base could be incorporated via either a problem-based approach or a client-based approach. For example in a problem-based approach where you take a presenting disorder such as dysphasia or in this scenario dysphagia, the key terms, presenting features and factors to consider in the assessment and management of the disorder can be presented. Teaching methods in this approach may include video presentations of dysphagic individuals or workshops involving role-play of assessments aimed at increasing the student's observational and decision-making skills, as well as enhancing self-awareness. Oropharyngeal assessments, for example, could be taught in workshops involving role-play. This component would also sit easily within the motor speech disorders module.

In a client-based approach, the focus will be on a particular client group such as stroke or neurodegenerative conditions. In this scenario, dysphagia can be incorporated by including case studies, for example of a client presenting with a stroke and dysphagia. This can allow exploration of taking a case history, identifying indicative features of dysphagia in this client group, and consideration of a plan of appropriate assessment techniques and management strategies.

In practice, the most successful way of adding the dysphagia knowledge base into the curricula is to integrate the two models.

The RCSLT document also states that graduates from a speech and language therapy qualifying course will have the practical competencies to be able to:

- carry out an assessment on a client with a non-complex condition to detect the presence or absence of dysphagia; this may include oropharyngeal examination, assessment of a dry swallow and trial of food consistencies
- make recommendations for management of a client with a non-complex condition
- consult and liaise with other members of the multidisciplinary team, including their speech and language therapist supervisor.

These skills can be taught in the pre-registration curriculum using a variety of methods. Simulation and role-play is one method. Simulation is a student-centred activity that aims to increase the students' understanding of others. It creates a safe environment where students may practise and improve on existing skills. The weakness of this method is the 'unreal' situation and absence of real dysphagic symptoms in the simulation activity.

Another method is that of demonstration. This is a teacher-centred activity which can utilize the students' previous experience in a safe environment. For example, the lecturer can demonstrate an oromotor assessment, the student can then practise the components while being supervised and the student can then go on to demonstrate the whole examination.

A difficulty that can become apparent in both these methods, however, is when the student lacks either the confidence or the interpersonal and social skills to practise the activity.

By the end of the pre-registration course the student is required to demonstrate the acquisition of these recommended skills. However, the RCSLT document accepts that there are variations in the practical clinical placements that individual students experience and it was not envisaged that every student would have a specialized dysphagia placement. The recommendation was clear that students should be given the opportunity to 'observe assessment procedures and a variety of treatment techniques, practise developing skills with normal subjects and assist with assessments/treatments where appropriate'.

In contrast, when the American Speech and Hearing Association proposed a curriculum for meeting the educational and workplace needs of graduate students, it suggested 4 hours of lecture time each week plus lab and clinical observations of 1–2 hours per week. Clinical observations were suggested as three cases, and observations were to include at least one instrumental evaluation, one non-instrumental evaluation and one treatment session and dysphagia team intervention. The graduate-level practical component is then suggested as 60 hours, which is to include diagnostic and treatment activities with an experienced clinician in a medical setting, nursing, special education or rehabilitation programme. Hence the US curriculum places a much greater emphasis on acquiring the practical competencies alongside the knowledge base.

Teaching competence

It can be argued that passing an examination in dysphagia does not give sufficient indication of practical competence. So how can training courses develop the practical skills of their students? How much learning gets transferred into clinical practice? Course attendance is surely not enough. Some learning theories are based on the concept that for learning to take place the individual has to engage actively in the experience and derive some meaning from it. Fish et al. (1991) argue that individuals need to know how to observe, analyse and consider critically what has been seen of an event or learning and refining will not occur. An individual needs to be able to reflect on what he or she has done or will do as a result. Observation and analysis skills can be acquired by using video recordings of patient assessment and treatment activities during teaching sessions. This method of teaching is an invaluable precursor to the student taking part in the activity with a live patient. The student can critically appraise the activity and discuss components of good and bad dysphagia practice, and can plan the next stages of the activity in a safe and controlled environment.

Eraut (1994) maintained, however, that the development of competence and expertise is inextricably linked to the context of practice. Using the formal pre-registration education programmes for student speech and language therapists to develop dysphagia knowledge and understanding undoubtedly has benefits for both the student and the speech and language therapy services that will be the future employers. The future employer would gain from not having to fund new therapists to attend further training courses soon after the start of their employment and would hope to be employing newly qualified therapists who have some skills in the area of dysphagia. However, the development of practical skills and competencies tends to be more effective if gained in the workplace and is related to individual patient needs. Therefore the acquisition of dysphagia skills and competencies would probably sit better in the therapists' development post-qualification and once they are within the working environment. This leads one then to ask whether there appears to be some discord between current university policy and the requirements of the employers, particularly with reference to the final examination system which satisfies academic standards rather than meeting employers' needs.

In Australia, competency-based occupational standards have been developed that include competencies within the field of dysphagia which entry level speech pathologists are expected to be able to demonstrate. These competencies include those for dysphagia in both developmental and acquired pathology disorders. Students tend to have a placement that is either specific to or has a large proportion of the time spent in acquiring the practical competency standards for dysphagia. Students are supervised by an experienced clinician and are assessed in the workplace by their supervisor in the acquisition of the practical competency standards, for example carrying out a bedside assessment of a patient. This is in contrast to the RCSLT document, which states that not all speech and language therapy students in Britain would have a placement specializing in dysphagia.

In comparison to the speech and language therapy student education the nursing profession in Britain focuses much more on practical ward-based learning opportunities. When student nurses are required to develop practical competencies in areas such as identifying tachycardia as opposed to the presence of a normal heart rate, they are taught the theory in the classroom environment but the practical competencies are achieved while on placement in the ward environment. Students observe an assessment, carry out the assessment under supervision and are then assessed carrying out the procedure themselves. To show competence, the student nurse is required to submit evidence of his or her ability to perform the assessment. This evidence may be in a learning log, shown through observed practice, demonstrated by being able to contextualize practice in reflective discussion or in the form of the supervisor obtaining the opinion of other assessors who have worked alongside the student. Hence the focus of student nurse training is much more embedded in the workplace and on learning in the real-life situation than traditional speech and language therapy pre-registration learning, which continues to have a greater focus on academic and classroom-based teaching.

The RCSLT paper recognizes that the objective of pre-registration dysphagia education and training should be to provide students with a basic level of competence to allow them to work in the field of dysphagia under the supervision of a more experienced clinician. However, in reality, many newly qualified clinicians experience difficulty accessing quality or even adequate on-site supervision, and the value of long-distance supervision, often over the telephone, is questionable. This may then lead to the newly qualified therapist and the client being exposed to an unacceptable level of risk.

The clinician working in the field of dysphagia is frequently required to make rapid decisions regarding a person's ability to eat and drink safely. Thomas Murry recognizes that 'both training and clinical experience often guide decision making' (Murry and Carrau, 2001). For newly qualified therapists, although these decisions may have a sound theoretical basis, they will not be made by clinicians with experience. Experience means having the ability to make the right use of knowledge. Alsop (1995) suggests that 'experience is a meaningful encounter, not just an observation. It is not passive, but an active engagement with the environment' and that 'experience stems from participation and not just from observation'.

Dysphagia is a complex problem, thus dealing with patients is a complex matter. There are numerous variables to consider and the balance of these may change for an individual over time as health status changes. Knowledge alone is not enough to deal effectively with these situations;

clinical reasoning and informed professional judgements are crucial. In moving this clinical field into the pre-registration arena and designing the dysphagia modules in the speech and language courses, how well was the question as to how these programmes would support the students' development of the required practical competencies necessary for working in such a complex and life-threatening area addressed and answered? Practising a new language assessment after gaining the theoretical knowledge can be both confusing and tricky, but does not carry the same risks as practising feeding techniques on a patient presenting with swallowing problems. In community settings, it is frequently difficult to access different members of the multidisciplinary team and gain timely support. How are pre-qualification courses addressing this risk issue with their students and how are they ensuring students have the required confidence and skills to minimize risk to their clients in these situations? In the document *Delivering Quality Care* (NHS Executive, 1998), it states that 'classroom and simulation based activities, whilst effective for developing knowledge and basic skills, are unlikely to develop true competence'. The real world of healthcare is dynamic and unpredictable, and healthcare professionals need to be competent to make careful risk assessments and to act on these appropriately without putting the client at further risk.

Placements for dysphagia

It is common knowledge that university pre-registration training courses are facing difficulties in finding enough suitable placements for their students, and clinical placement tutors are having to work with practising clinicians to find novel ways of approaching placements. It has been recognized that the main limiting factor in meeting the government's aim to increase student numbers is the lack of clinical placements offered by the profession as a whole (Rossiter, 2001). Therefore, adding dysphagia to the numerous practical requirements it is necessary for the student to experience is surely not sensible. It was argued by some clinicians at the time that once dysphagia was accepted onto the curriculum, placements in acute hospitals, which had been lost to students because of the focus on dysphagia, would then become open to them again.

In reality, however, can a student gain enough practical dysphagia competencies in such a short period of time to make them 'fit-for-purpose' to the employer? Pre-requisite skills to the hands-on assessment and management of dysphagia can, however, be successfully gained during the current clinical placement periods. For example, the skills in assessing a patient's cognitive and linguistic status, which it is necessary for the clinician to know before deciding on and implementing an effective management plan for dysphagia; also, some of the skills required to assess a patient's physical and emotional status. Skills in gaining team awareness and professional networks are also fundamental, as are those of inter-personal communication between the student, client, carer and the rest of the team. Students need to be able to develop rapport with an individual in order to respond to and discuss the issues of dysphagia in a sensitive and empathic manner. They need to develop the skills of reflective questioning so they can elicit a case history and they need to be able to respond to both verbal and non-verbal indicators using appropriate communication techniques. If one focuses only on the component parts of performance there is a danger that the complexity and subtlety of the speech and language therapist's work may be lost. It is only with the integration and application of the knowledge base, practical skills and attitudes that professional performance becomes competent (Speech Pathology Association of Australia, 2001).

A further concern highlighted by clinicians is that by adding specific dysphagia competencies to those already expected to be gained in the clinical placements there must surely be a reduction in the exposure to communication-impaired patients. If components are added to the required knowledge base and skills without adding extra time to the academic year in which to gain these skills, then something else must be dropped from the curriculum or the issue becomes one of breadth of competency acquired versus depth of the competency. Placement time is already short and some educators and practising clinicians think the curriculum content is already overstretched.

Eraut (1994) suggested that the initial period in which novice professionals develop their proficiency in the general professional role continues well beyond their initial qualification, with the first two or three years post-qualification being the most influential. Clinical reasoning, with its reliance on experience, analogy and extrapolation, must be applied in the assessment and management of a client with dysphagia. At times, a decision may be contrary to evidence of effectiveness from the literature but may provide a more desirable outcome for the client. Are speech and language therapy students and newly qualified therapists equipped to deal with these dilemmas? This raises the issue as to where and even whether dysphagia knowledge and skills fit within the pre-registration course. The knowledge base sits comfortably within the curriculum, probably from year 1, when normal anatomy, physiology and neurology are incorporated. The dysphagia knowledge base does not need to be a separate module; it can be flagged or marked in some way by the individual lecturers as a component of the original course topic areas. It may also be useful for students to have at least a few hours during their final year to pull the component parts together in order to consider and raise the complex issues which are omnipresent when assessing and managing clients with dysphagia. It is the acquisition of the practical competencies and the components of clinical reasoning and judgement that appear to fit less clearly.

As in most fields of work of the practising speech and language therapist, there are no rigid directives or cookbook fixes in the field of dysphagia. It is hoped that clinicians will make 'recommendations that suit the safety needs of the patient tempered with a healthy respect for the innumerable combinations of health status elements, including quality of life, that can affect positive and negative outcomes' (Murray, 1999). Successful management of dysphagic patients requires knowledge of a range of technological developments, such as artificial nutrition and hydration, which prolong life but do not in themselves reverse a patient's disease. Hence patients with deteriorating conditions such as motor neurone disease may have their lives extended with artificial nutrition but their irreversible medical condition will eventually result in their death. Even the most experienced health professionals are known to feel anxiety and have emotional debates about when to offer treatments in life and death situations.

The ethical implications

Barnitt (1993), an educator in occupational therapy, asked both students and clinicians from occupational and physiotherapy 'what gives you sleepless nights?' Many of the responses revolved around issues to do with ethics and morals. Both the students and their clinical colleagues revealed feelings of inadequacy when faced with moral problems. The area of dysphagia is fraught with ethical and moral dilemmas, for example research suggests that the clinical bedside assessment misses 40% of patients who aspirate. However, many services have limited access to more objective assessments for their patients. A further example is when a patient is assessed and determined as having a swallow mechanism that is unable to cope safely with oral food and drink; however, it is not always the case that the patient should be fed by alternative feeding methods. The patient's quality of life is paramount. Eating and drinking are fundamental biological processes and being denied this simple and basic drive to satisfy thirst and hunger can be both demeaning and demoralizing for the patient (Murray, 1999). A high level of skill is required to deal holistically with these dilemmas.

There is often no single correct answer to an ethical or moral dilemma and the individual therapist has to carry out a thorough reasoning process to arrive at the best possible outcome. Students could be taught the general ethical principles involved in dysphagia care alongside medical ethics. Case scenarios could be presented for small group discussion so that issues are well debated and thus equip students with some of the moral arguments. The case scenarios could, for example, be used to address the issue of feeding a patient even though he or she is at risk of aspiration, or the issue of feeding a patient by alternative means when he or she is in the terminal stages of a disease process.

Moral decision making is thought of as a developmental process by which a therapist learns to reason about a topic. Barnitt recognizes that 'ethics is not a subject that can be taught like anatomy ... it requires a process of careful deliberation. While the end product may be unknown and cannot be gauged in terms of correctness, the reasoning task that has been used to arrive at the end point is the important skill.' This raises the question as to whether pre-registration courses are able to address successfully the issue of day-to-day ethics practised by the therapist.

Barnitt's study found that the therapists interviewed were 'on the whole very clear about their moral rules and skilled at supporting their beliefs. Problems for the therapists usually arose where their moral rule was challenged by the client or other members of the treatment team.' This scenario is not uncommon in the field of dysphagia working. The ethics around dysphagia and its management are known to be particularly challenging even for the most experienced clinicians because they contrast scientific approaches with health and wellbeing. Therefore again it is necessary to ask the question, whether we are expecting too much of newly qualified therapists in the profession if we require them to have the knowledge and skills to work with this life-threatening condition so early on in their career development.

Learning about competence: legal implications

One component of professional competence that could become critical relates to the scope of practice for newly qualified speech and language therapists. The RCSLT Code of Ethics and Professional Conduct states that speech and language therapists should 'operate within the parameters of their own competence' and clinicians are expected to offer interventions that maximize benefit and minimize harm to their clients (Alsop, 1997). Extending the scope of practice of newly trained speech and language therapists should be considered carefully and be the subject of prudent scrutiny and robust research, particularly as dysphagia is considered to be one of the most stressful and contentious conditions managed by speech and language therapists (Dawson et al., 1996).

Their article published in the *Australian Communication Quarterly* describes a process where newly qualified speech and language therapists were interviewed to determine incidents that they found particularly unsuccessful or stressful. Out of 46 incidents, 32% concerned the management of dysphagia. Examples were given where, for instance, 'a typical stressful situation involving dysphagia was one where the speech pathologist, who was in a locum position, was asked to assess the swallowing of a tracheotomized client on an intensive care ward'. Other examples cited include situations where the new speech pathologist's authority was challenged by staff or relatives, for example: 'A speech pathologist had made a recommendation that a client be nil-by-mouth and be fed by a nasogastric tube because of clearly observable aspiration. However, the client pulled the naso-gastric tube out, which led to the speech pathologist's recommendations being questioned.'

Up to now it has been extremely rare for speech and language therapists to be sued for negligence, but in an increasingly litigious society it is surely only a matter of time (Horner, 1999). It must be remembered that the clinician needs to sleep at night and frequent recounting of the day's decisions and recommendations to his or her clients and carers is not conducive to a good night's sleep. The person suing will remember the events very clearly because it has been central to his or her life. The clinician, on the other hand, may struggle to recall the precise words used and recommendations given. The judge will decide the case on the balance of probabilities and who has produced the best evidence. However, if the clinician has acted professionally and recorded these actions accordingly, then he or she is not at risk. Speech and language therapists 'must work without fear or favour, in the best interests of the client, acting on behalf of the employer, striving to uphold professional standards and maintaining the trust that society has placed in them. That way they have nothing to fear. The responsibility, however, is nobody's but theirs' (Andrews and Wheeler, 1996). Are we therefore expecting too much from novice speech and language therapists, who are already grappling with the challenges of working life, and are they suitably equipped to manage a client with a life-threatening condition at this stage of their careers and professional development? One of the important responsibilities of newly qualified speech and language therapists is for them to recognize when they do not know something and when to ask for help and support. Experienced clinicians may find it easy to ask for help, but often for new clinicians, asking for help or admitting lack of knowledge may exacerbate any feelings of inadequacy or of not being seen to successfully cope and manage their clients.

Current educational theory accepts that, with the explosion in information, it is impossible to include all relevant information in a crowded curriculum. Recently, newly qualified therapists have been encouraged to think of their speech and language therapy qualification as a first step in the process of lifelong learning and professional development. For clinical educators and service managers it may require a reconsideration of whether dysphagia competencies are realistic skills for newly qualified therapists or whether they are better acquired later in the clinician's professional development. Successful management of a dysphagic client requires not only the ability to draw from knowledge and practical skills, but also the ability to draw from ethical knowledge and the ability to take a holistic view of the client and the prognostic variables. Although these areas begin to be addressed at a pre-registration level are they developed sufficiently to equip the newly registered therapist to deal with a dysphagic caseload?

This leads one to ask what criteria would result in the judgement of a student 'failing' in dysphagia competence. In my experience of training post-qualification therapists, it is often not the ability to perform the task, for example carrying out an oropharyngeal swallowing assessment, that is the problem, but the clinician's inability to develop rationale or use adequate clinical reasoning. Often it is the clinician's lack of ability to reflect and make sound clinical judgements based on clear and effective reasoning that results in him or her being deemed incompetent. Some students do not find this an easy process to carry through into practice and only develop the skill through further ongoing well-supervised practice in the workplace, and this can, in some cases, take many hours to achieve.

New initiatives: an alternative approach

An alternative approach to training pre-registration speech and language therapy students in the competencies of dysphagia assessment and management can be drawn from the new initiatives in the NHS, which demand more partnership and collaborative working to develop services that are integrated at the point of delivery and which have at their centre the needs of the patient. The *NHS Plan* (DoH, 2000a) and the *National Service Framework* (NSF) *for Older People* (DoH, 2001) have key implications for the roles of professionals and the need for sharing of specialist skills with their nursing colleagues. The *Comprehensive Critical Care* document (DoH, 2000b) stresses the importance of sharing critical care skills such as dysphagia across the team, particularly as critical care is a 24-hours-a-day, seven-days-a-week service. The document *Critical to Success* (Audit Commission, 2001), states that it is imperative for training to be rolled out to ward staff to help prevent admissions to critical care beds. It is now becoming increasingly obvious to many speech and language therapists that total reliance on our service to provide assessments of the safety of patients' swallowing puts enormous strain on both individual therapists and resources and does not provide the best service to the patients.

One answer is to move away from the traditional pattern of only speech and language therapists being trained and responsible for providing dysphagia assessment and management, and moving towards a more responsive and flexible service where selected nurses are trained in the theoretical and practical competencies to allow them to work alongside their local speech and language therapy colleagues. This vision requires new thinking about the delivery of dysphagia services and is based on:

- interdisciplinary working and skill sharing while still recognizing different professional needs and boundaries
- providing readily accessible, responsive and flexible services
- providing appropriate education, training and support across professions
- putting the patient at the centre of care.

According to the Royal College of Nursing (RCN, 1996), 'Nurses have traditionally played a key, practical role in meeting the nutritional needs of hospital patients.' The RCN states that the responsibilities of nurses should be to ensure that:

- patients' nutritional needs are met
- patients' preferences for particular foods are identified, especially where this is influenced by religious, cultural or ethnic reasons
- patients are sitting or lying in a position so that they can reach drinks and eat their food
- patients do not have dental problems, in particular that dentures fit properly and are in use
- where necessary, patients have special equipment to help them eat
- patients have no problems eating, for example, whether or not they are finding it difficult to swallow or have any mouth infections which would affect their ability to eat.

The RCSLT (1999) states that:

- Speech and language therapists possess a sound knowledge of the structure and function of the vocal tract. They are skilled in the assessment and remediation of voice and speech disorders arising from neurological, structural and psychological aetiologies.
- Knowledge and skills developed in this area have been extended and applied to assessment, intervention and management of clients with dysphagia.
- The College supports the principle that speech and language therapists as a professional group are ideally equipped to take a central role within the multidisciplinary team in the assessment and remediation of swallowing disorders.
- The aims of a dysphagia service are to:
  - provide a comprehensive and responsive service to clients presenting with eating and swallowing disorders
  - facilitate intervention as part of the multidisciplinary team
  - become engaged in the planning of services to potential clients presenting with eating and swallowing disorders.

The two professional groups need to consider their individual roles and 'blur' the boundaries while still recognizing each other's unique contribution. They need to reassess and remodel traditional roles, with the aim of nurses working in partnership with their speech and language therapy colleagues and thus creating a multiskilled workforce trained to deliver better and more cost-effective patient services.

The complex nature of dysphagia means patients should be managed on a team basis, where the team is working in partnership, thus ensuring that the dysphagic patient receives careful, in-depth assessment and treatment of the swallowing disorder and its underlying aetiology. Team members need to respect each other's expertise and communicate quickly and easily with each other. The method of communication is less important than the quality of the communication. The quality of the patient experience, as well as the clinical result, is a fundamental component of better care, that is quality should be measured in terms not only of prompt access but also good relationships and communication between the healthcare team and the client. A therapist needs to be confident in his or her own knowledge and skills in order to work as a full team player and to be able to share skills successfully. Newly qualified therapists need time to consolidate their own identity and role as professionals before they are able to work effectively in dysphagia partnerships.

The Department of Health publication *Future Staffing Requirements* (DoH, 1999) states that: 'the Government recognises the importance of multidisciplinary education and training as a means of developing and promoting effective team working and integrated care. The research has shown that:

- there is a perception that multidisciplinary education fosters and enhances collaborative working practices
- integrated workforce planning is a significant driver for the development of multidisciplinary education
- multidisciplinary education supports changes in patterns of service delivery and
- it is perceived to be more effective at post registration level than at pre-registration level.'

Within the field of dysphagia we should therefore be exploring opportunities for shared learning at both pre-registration and post-registration levels. For example at pre-registration level, it is not uncommon for first-year speech and language therapy students to have their anatomy and physiology lectures alongside medical students. This concept of joint learning could be expanded later on in the course and would then begin to break down professional boundaries and establish shared values. For example, at pre-registration level, it would be valuable for students to attend joint medical ethic workshops with medical, nursing and other allied health professional students. This would widen the debate and identify and share cross-professional views and perspectives before the speech and language therapy students and their future colleagues are expected to work in the real context.

Learning in the workplace as part of a multidisciplinary team, across professional and service boundaries is becoming increasingly important and is where approaches to teaching dysphagia should be heading in the future.

At a post-registration level, joint learning in workshops would allow dysphagia to be explored as a part of many professional roles rather than seeing it as a task that is within the remit of the speech and language therapy profession only. For instance, exploring the complex issues which affect dysphagic patients on a ward or in a nursing home with all the professional groups involved may lead to greater compliance with recommendations for dietary changes or postural changes to enhance safe swallowing or to increase the patient's nutritional intake.

Developing better quality and more responsive services for dysphagic patients means developing new approaches to healthcare and the training and education of healthcare staff. Successful partnerships at local and national level will be essential if these innovative approaches are to succeed. This will need to include individual professionals and their managers, professional associations, and educational providers and commissioners. The expertise of the professional bodies will need to support the approach to the sharing of the role within the context of clinical governance. Service and education partnerships will need to be created in order to design and deliver flexible, modular education and training in the dysphagia knowledge base, and the practical competencies of assessment and management of dysphagia. Uniprofessional training should continue to play an important part in the establishment of each profession's unique and core skills, perhaps at the pre-registration level. However, there is equally a need to build a culture of shared values to allow the development of shared knowledge, skills and competencies, perhaps at a post-registration level. This will result in more effective partnership working across traditional professional boundaries and should result in a more responsive and better quality service for the dysphagic client. However, until the speech and language therapy profession is able to determine the competencies required along the dysphagia continuum for clinicians at different stages of their professional and career development, the provision by educational establishments of appropriate theoretical knowledge and practical competencies will remain unclear and ambiguous.

References

Alsop A (1995) The professional portfolio – purpose, process and practice, Part 2: Producing a portfolio from experiential learning. British Journal of Occupational Therapy 58: 337–340.

Alsop A (1997) Evidence based practice and continuing professional development. British Journal of Occupational Therapy 60: 503–507.

Andrews A, Wheeler N (1996) Accountability and occupational therapy. British Journal of Occupational Therapy 59: 483–484.

Audit Commission (2001) Critical to Success. London: Audit Commission.

Barnitt R (1993) What gives you sleepless nights? Ethical practice in occupational therapy. British Journal of Occupational Therapy 56: 207–212.

Bright M (1997) She was dying for a cuppa. Literally. The Observer 1 April.

Dawson V, Cichero J, Pattie M (1996) When to ask for help – the base-grade speech pathologist working in dysphagia: an interpretation of the competency-based occupational standards and the dysphagia position paper. Australian Communication Quarterly Spring: 4–6.

Dobinson S, Parr C (1991) Therapists feelings about working with dysphagic people. RCSLT Bulletin 473: 6–7.

DoH (1999) Future Staffing Requirements. London: Department of Health.

DoH (2000a) The NHS Plan. London: Department of Health.

DoH (2000b) Comprehensive Critical Care. A Review of Adult Critical Care Services. London: Department of Health.

DoH (2001) National Service Framework for Older People. London: Department of Health.

Eraut M (1994) Developing Professional Knowledge and Competence. London: Falmer Press

Fish D, Twinn S, Purr B (1991) Promoting Reflection: Improving the Supervision of Practice in Health Visiting and Teacher Training. Isleworth, Middlesex: West London Institute of Higher Education.

Giles J, Davison A (1996) SLT and nursing: partners in dysphagia. RCSLT Bulletin December: 10–11.

Health Advisory Service (1998) Not Because They're Old. London: Department of Health.

Horner S (1999) Dysphagia dilemma: an issue of clinical governance. RCSLT Bulletin 566: 16.

Kohler ES (1991) A dysphagia management model for rural elderly. Physical and Occupational Therapy in Geriatrics 10: 81–94.

Murray J (1999) Manual of Dysphagia Assessment in Adults. San Diego, CA: Singular Publishing Group.

Murry T, Carrau R (2001) Clinical Manual for Swallowing Disorders. San Diego, CA: Singular Publishing Group.

NHS Executive (1998) Delivering Quality Care. Leeds: Department of Health.

Odderson R, Keaton JC, McKenna BS (1995) Swallow management in patients on an acute stroke pathway: quality is cost effective. Archives of Physical Medicine Rehabilitation 76: 1130–1133.

O'Leary I (1991)Who should be working on dysphagia? RCSLT Bulletin 470: 7.

O'Loughlin G, Shanley C (1998) Swallowing problems in the nursing home: a novel training response. Dysphagia 13:172–183.

RCN (1996) RCN Statement on Feeding and Nutrition in Hospitals. London: Royal College of Nursing.

RCSLT (1996) Communicating Quality 2: Professional Standards for Speech and Language Therapists, 2nd edn. London: Royal College of Speech and Language Therapists.

RCSLT Advanced Studies Committee Dysphagia Working Group (1999) Recommendations for Pre- and Post-registration Dysphagia Education and Training. London: Royal College of Speech and Language Therapists.

Rossiter D (2001) Student placements: the whole profession's responsibility. RCSLT Bulletin 594: 4.

Scottish Intercollegiate Guidelines Network. Pilot Edition (1997) Management of Patients with Stroke. Identification and Management of Dysphagia. Edinburgh: Scottish Intercollegiate Guidelines Network.

Speech Pathology Association of Australia (2001) Competency Based Occupational Standards for Speech Pathology – Entry Level. Melbourne: Speech Pathology Association of Australia.

White G, Whitaker J, David R, Wright J, Hughes G, Syder D (1993) Forum produces dysphagia action plan. CSLT Bulletin 490: 4–5.

Chapter 6
Fit for practice: new models for clinical placements

Sue Baxter

Introduction

This chapter discusses the necessity for clinical education to revisit the traditional workplace placement models that have educated students since the professions began. As education has shifted its emphasis from being teacher-centred to being learner-centred, and as adult education has been recognized as a distinct field from education in schools, there has been a huge growth in the literature available to inform clinical education. There is a need for the education of professionals to further develop as an area of study, building on the work in adult and higher education, to become a recognized field in its own right.

The education of professionals to work in clinical environments has undergone a huge shift, following the change in funding of health professional training in the UK, from the local authority to National Health Service bursaries. The education providers are now not only in a relationship with the professional bodies, but also with the workforce confederations who decide number of students in training and issue contracts, while maintaining their position within the university institutions. These changes in funding have caused professional education to become increasingly under the spotlight, with workplace experience being given more recognition than simply the place where theory is applied. Changes in the working practices of the professions and the need to prepare students to practise in an ever-changing working environment have also meant a re-examinination of clinical education. The time is therefore nigh for an examination of current clinical teaching methods, to use the available literature to inform and extend best practice.

Traditional placement models

For students, the clinical placement aspects of a course tend to be the most remembered and influential experiences of their training. Ask any professional, and he or she will be able to recount tales of his or her clinical placements – both good and not so good. It is often these remembered experiences that shape how a professional responds to the challenge of taking students on clinical placement. The models that have traditionally been used can make several assumptions.

- That theory should be taught by the training institute and precede practice.
- That learners should observe an experienced practitioner for some time before trying it out themselves.
- That learners should either be observed by the practitioner at all times or alternatively should be 'left to get on with it'.
- That one student should be placed with one practitioner.
- That students are given whichever placements are available.
- That placement hours are spent with practising clinicians from their chosen discipline.

These assumptions are discussed below, and the literature on professional education is used to inform these areas, suggesting new models for clinical placements. The chapter concludes with an outline of three models of placement provision that have been developed, which draw on the literature and offer the possibility of new ways forward.

Theory and practice

In the field of higher education, 'applied' courses have traditionally been accorded lower status than those that are 'pure' knowledge based. For this reason it has seemed that clinical courses have worked hard to ensure the 'theory' components of the course have been given primary recognition over 'practice'. In the curriculum of most courses there was the expectation that students would spend the initial phases absorbing themselves in the theoretical aspects, for example learning anatomy and physiology, linguistics, psychology, and sociology. Once the students were grounded in these disciplines they would then go out to the workplace and naturally 'apply' their learning. In recent years, many courses have recognized the rather artificial distinction created by learning via this route and have begun to adopt approaches that have attempted to encourage transferability in learning between knowledge from different disciplines. Problem-based learning (see, for example, Boud and Feletti, 1991) is one such method, where the focus is in on a clinical problem and possible solutions using all available information. A second option adopted by some training courses is to revise the curriculum to create learning 'tracks' covering information relevant to a topic from all fields.

An important model for looking at clinical education has been the knowledge, skills, attitude paradigm (see, for example, Stenglehoffen, 1993) drawing on the behaviour dimensions of cognitive, motor and affective. This framework has been an extremely useful one in professional training, helping to identify exactly what areas need to be acquired to become a competent practitioner. It has been used successfully to form the basis of assessment tools. However, the difficulty lies in making some of the aspects observable and measurable, particularly when it comes to attitude. The model continues to be widely used, but can be criticized for failing to take sufficient account of the interplay between factors, and although its strength is in its clarity and simplicity, the real situation in clinical training tends to be more interwoven and complex.

Some writers have highlighted what they see as the artificial gap between knowledge, skills and attitude or 'theory' and 'practice'. Carr and Kemmis (1986: 112) drew attention to the fact that 'theory' is a notion that can be used in a variety of ways. It can refer to causal explanations used in disciplines, or it can refer to general frameworks that are used in practice. Thus theory is not distinct from practice as 'all theories are the product of some practical activity, so all practical activities are guided by some theory' (Carr and Kemmis 1986: 113). Dreyfus and Dreyfus (1986: 17) also integrate theory and practice into a distinction between 'knowing how' and 'knowing that'. The 'knowing that' can refer to facts and rules, but the 'knowing how' is acquired from practice. They believed it was possible to identify five stages in the process of moving from a novice to an expert, from 'knowing that' to 'knowing how'. These stages record the development of a professional from being able to deal in an analytical way with structured problems, to being able to deal with unstructured problems in an almost intuitive way.

This view of knowledge and practice being bound up together has been further explored through the work of Schon (1983) and Argyris and Schon (1991). They drew attention to the difference between 'espoused theory' and 'theory-in-use'. 'Espoused theories' are the initially learned theories, the theories within disciplines. The 'theories-in-use', however, are governed by an individual's attitudes, values and beliefs. The individual receiving information will adapt and amend the 'received wisdom', incorporating it into his or her own 'theory-in-use', which governs practice. Michael Eraut (1994) further extended this work into his proposal of professional knowledge as consisting of three different elements (see Introduction, page xv). First, there is process knowledge, which refers to knowing how to conduct practice. Second, there is personal knowledge, which refers to the individual's beliefs and attitudes. Finally, there is propositional knowledge, which is the discipline-based knowledge; this is the aspect usually perceived to be the 'theory' element of a course. Eraut reminds us, however, that even in this aspect, propositional knowledge 'cannot be characterised in a manner that is independent of how it is learned and how it is used' (Eraut 1994: 45). It is not accurate to think of theory learned and then applied to practice, as the knowledge changes in its use.

So how should this work inform clinical training and clinical placement models? First, it seems that the divide between 'theory' and 'practice' should be seen as an artificial one; there is a need for the 'theories-in-use' that students are exposed to by being with practising clinicians to be verbalized in order to be understood by the student. It is important that clinicians do not view themselves as simply the provider of the 'practice component', but recognize the dynamic interaction between knowledge and practice. Clinicians should recognize their wealth of 'theory-in-use' knowledge. Clinicians often say 'I don't really use any theory in my day-to-day working'; their theory has become so implicit that they have lost the awareness of it. They have reached Dreyfus and Dreyfus's level of 'expert', using clinical intuition (the area of practice Schon (1983) called 'professional artistry'). By clinicians attempting to make visible these areas of practice through discussion of clinical decision making and reasoning behind actions, students can begin to construct their own 'knowledge-in-use'.

By removing the old theory/practice divisions and looking at knowledge acquisition in different ways, the old model of students being given all the theory before they learn to 'apply it', seems out of step with reality. Newer models of clinical education are incorporating clinical work much earlier into training, and encouraging students to access the knowledge required to support clinical learning, rather than clinical learning being used to apply knowledge. The recognition that in the modern world, factual knowledge has only a limited 'shelf life' has also encouraged a shift from learning 'what' to learning 'how to find out'. Students need to develop process knowledge of learning how to manage information, how to update knowledge and how to access literature databases. The propositional knowledge of today may be outdated in a few years time. Clinical placements need to foster that process of information gathering and updating, encouraging students to find out information for themselves, and debate the merits of current theory, offering alternative perspectives rather than 'pure facts'. This need for clinical placements to offer active seeking of information will be further explored as an aspect of independent learning.

Observation and practice

Traditional models of clinical placement have offered students 'observation' placements in the early stages of training, before they were ready and able to take on 'hands-on' experience. This often meant students sitting in the corner of a clinic watching the session and, if there was time afterwards, the clinician talking through what was going on. Most practising clinicians today will have experienced these passive observation sessions, clearly remembering the desperate struggle to stay awake and look interested. This learning experience is described by one of my colleagues as the 'sitting next to Nellie' approach. The student enters the learning environment, sits in the presence of the therapist and by some process akin to osmosis is able to perform in the same way as the clinician when that stage of the course arrives. It is hoped that this model is a rare occurrence nowadays, but the likelihood is that it still exists.

The literature on adult learning has encouraged a move away from this passive learning experience into a more self-directed active model. The need to involve learners more in their learning grew originally from the humanist movement, particularly the work of Carl Rogers in the 1970s. Mezirow (1983) emphasized the importance of critical reflection in the learning process; in order to maximize learning from the experience. This was further explored and extended by Boud et al. (1993), who recognized the importance of students taking the responsibility for their own learning in a self-directed learning approach. Boud (1988) suggested a continuum of dependence, from independence to interdependence, as a student becomes less reliant on a practitioner. He emphasized that a student being presented with a learning experience does not automatically ensure learning takes place, he felt that it was a process of reflection during or after the learning experience that led to learning.

In the literature, terms such as 'self-directed learning', 'independent learning' and 'active learning' seem to be used almost interchangeably. Taylor (1997) feels that 'independent learning' is the most appropriate term in professional education, as students are required to be able to operate both independently and interdependently in practice. 'Self-directed learning' implies little interaction between a student and other learners, or a learner and more experienced colleagues. It is important that students learn to work collaboratively with colleagues and seek help and guidance when required, working independently but also interdependently. Taylor (1997) offers an important reminder that students need orientation to this method of learning, as it can challenge many of a learner's assumptions about teaching and learning. It should not be assumed that students are immediately able to utilize this learning approach without guidance.

As mentioned above, along with the notion of students taking responsibility for their own learning, the place of reflection in the learning cycle has also assumed increasing importance. Lincoln et al. (1997a: 101) state that 'reflective practice helps students make sense of their experiences, and become competent practitioners. It is the responsibility of educators therefore to provide students with strategies to facilitate reflective practice.' They go on to outline useful methods of fostering reflection through journal writing, video feedback and conferences.

So what principles should be taken to inform clinical placement provision? First, placements should recognize the importance of students being actively involved in the learning. Many training establishments are questioning the value of 'observational' placements, particularly early on in the course when the students have no experience to inform their observations. The literature emphasizes the importance of experience being the key to learning, but without a reflective component in the learning the value is lessened.

The role of the supervisor

For some students the first time they have worked with a patient without a supervising clinician present is their first day as a qualified practitioner. Morris (2001) explored access to learning for speech and language therapy students in terms of risk management. In the study, clinicians reported their concerns regarding the wellbeing of clients and students, as well as the risks posed to the service by students being allowed access to clients without qualified staff present. So what should a clinical teacher do? Parsell and Bligh (2001) refer to effective clinical teaching as being 'complex and multidimensional'. They identify four main roles of a clinical teacher, as: physician (clinical expert), teacher, supervisor and supporter. They emphasize that these roles change as the student becomes more independent, proficient and skilled. The importance of students becoming independent and interdependent is a key concept again here.

As students will be working in a rapidly changing world, in their role as 'a professional' they will be expected to have a degree of autonomy. It is vital that students develop to be reflective assessors of their own practice and able to operate independently. To achieve this it is essential that students experience some autonomy during the latter stages of training and view themselves as 'professionals in training' rather than 'a student'. Few of us behave naturally when we know that we are under observation and every wrong word will be fed back following the session. Who would not look to a supervising clinician for help, if one were present, when they got stuck? It is not easy for clinicians to see a student making an error without 'leaping in' to correct it. The process of students moving from student to practitioner is poorly documented. Ewan (1988) refers to the process of becoming a professional as 'professional socialization', believing it to be part of a hidden curriculum in most courses. It seems that students become professionals at some point before graduation, but it is not specified when or how. Lincoln et al. (1997b) also emphasize the importance of professionalism, asserting that students 'do not become professionals simply by learning theory or completing clinical experience' (Lincoln et al., 1997b: 76). They identify four elements of professionalism: technical competence, professional interpersonal skills, knowledge of professional standards of conduct and ethical competence.

It is important to recognize that the role of the supervisor is not fixed. It can change from student to student and between situations. The student should be allowed the chance to be an independent learner, appropriate for his or her stage of training and taking risk factors into account. For students to become practising professionals, the issues of becoming a professional need to become transparent and students need to be given the opportunity to develop these skills. Clearly a supervisor who is permanently absent is providing ample opportunity for the student to learn professional responsibility, but is giving little feedback on learning or chance for the student to seek support and guidance when required. However, the student who never experiences working without the supervisor present and never has to 'think on their feet' risks remaining dependent and experiencing a traumatic launch into practice.

Individual versus peer learning

As this has been covered in depth in Chapter 3, this chapter will only briefly echo the importance and benefits of this approach. Students learning on placement with other students offer considerable support and the opportunity to seek clarification between themselves regarding any uncertainties. Students benefit considerably from their early clinical experience being with other students, as they are able to compare their abilities to their peers, rather than to an experienced, practising clinician. As will be discussed further, there is now a considerable demand to train practitioners who are capable of working in multidisciplinary teams. There is evidence emerging from the literature that learning to work in unidisciplinary groups could be an important precursor to being able to work with other professionals (Barr et al., 2000; Smith et al., 1996). Teamworking skills, whether unidisciplinary or multidisciplinary, are an essential requirement for today's practitioners. Students need to learn to work cooperatively and collaboratively with peers, and small group working is now a regular part of university-based work. It is important, however, that these principles are extended into the clinical practice elements of a course and learning in pairs and groups needs to be part of the placement experience. As Barr (2000) states, 'work-based interprofessional education is much more likely than university-based education to result directly in changes in practice'.

Equity of experience

The clinical placement element of courses is usually provided in workplace settings, away from the training establishment. The requirement for the student in terms of hours of placement and client groups is usually stipulated, together with aims and objectives for the placement. The actual experience that the student receives is determined by the placement provider, and in these days of extreme shortages of placements, any offers received by a training establishment to take a student on placement are usually welcomed with open arms. Where students are placed for periods of weeks, on blocks, it is harder for training institutions and the placement providers themselves to guarantee in advance exactly what experiences the student will receive. With the formation of individual trusts, there is increasing local control over health service provision, and growing variation between service policies and provision across the country. Students therefore can experience very different learning opportunities and be exposed to different views of 'best practice'. This can provide for rich discussion when the students return to the training establishment, but can also raise issues for the course provider and NHS as placement provider if students are unhappy with the experience they have received.

As the student's rights as a 'consumer' come to the fore, with the prospects of litigation becoming less distant, equity of experience has become a real issue for the training providers. One way that can alleviate this difficulty is for the training establishments to work with local services to provide pre-determined, 'packaged' placement experiences, which are available to all students. There is also a need to reconsider whether placement hours are a sufficient measure of students' learning during a course. As education has shifted from an emphasis on what has been taught to what has been learned, it is surely time for professional bodies to look again at the requirement for registration to practice. The present measure of placement hours completed surely is an insufficient measure, and needs to be replaced by a log of experience and learning, or recognition of what skills/knowledge/personal qualities are required. In the UK, the RCSLT is engaged in a considerable task of establishing professional competencies, which needs to feed through as a continuum from initial education to continuing professional education.

Interprofessional learning

Currently, student placement hours in speech and language therapy are required to be under the supervision of a qualified speech and language therapist. With the increasing trend towards interprofessional course designs this may prove to be a challenging issue. Recent government policy documents have all emphasized the drive towards interprofessional learning and working. *The NHS Plan* (DoH, 2000a) emphasizes the need to promote multiprofessional working, and *Meeting the Challenge: A Strategy for the Allied Health Professionals* (DoH, 2000b) emphasizes that 'learning together can deliver added value for practitioners through developing an understanding of the roles of other professionals and building team working skills'. According to Barr et al. (2000), interprofessional education is reputed to: enhance motivation to collaborate, change attitudes and perception, cultivate interpersonal and group relations, and establish common values and knowledge bases. The ultimate aim, however, which sometimes seem to be forgotten in the general enthusiasm for interprofessional learning, is that interprofessional education should 'facilitate collaborative practice to improve the quality of patient care' (Barr, 2000). As Lowry et al. (2000) remind us, the client should always be the focus.

In the general government-led push towards interprofessional education, there is a growing literature with the aim of evaluating whether or not this offers the best way forward for professional education, and what exactly is achieved by educating professionals together. The area is not helped by the considerable confusion in terminology, between multiprofessional, interprofessional, multidisciplinary, interdisciplinary and shared learning, a confusion called a 'terminological quagmire' by Leathard (1994). It is vital that this terminology is clarified in order to compare the work of different authors, and as Finch (2000) pleads, 'without a clear definition of the desired interprofessional working practices, higher education cannot develop the pedagogical approaches which underpin it'. Finch feels there are four possible interpretations of what the NHS requires students to do. First, that they should know about the roles of other professional groups; second, that they should be able to work with other professionals as part of a team; third, that they should be able to substitute for other professionals, ending the old demarcation lines of role responsibility; and finally, that there should be flexibility in career routes, so that students can move between training courses.

It is not possible here to provide a complete and in-depth discussion of the work being carried out in this area. See Barr et al. (2000) for a comprehensive summary of the area, and Miller et al. (2001) for insightful discussions of the area and the way forward. For the purposes of this exploration of clinical placements it is sufficient to recognize the influence of work in the area and the growing importance of students graduating with the ability to work in teams with other professional groups. Miller et al. (2001) offer a useful summary of their proposals for the future of initial education of practitioners. First, they emphasize the difference between 'shared learning' and 'common learning'. 'Shared learning' refers to experiences where students learn with and from each other, which is very different from a 'common learning' agenda, where groups of students are taught together, giving a common knowledge base. This is a crucial distinction to draw, as many people's view of interprofessional learning is of common learning, which the literature suggests is of limited value. Miller et al. argue strongly that it is shared learning that maximizes the 'value added' by students learning together.

The second of Miller et al.'s proposals for interprofessional learning is that teamwork is the vital element to the delivery of health and social care, and that learning programmes need to provide experiences that build these skills. Third, they emphasize that interprofessional learning should be patient/client-focused, and recognize the changing status of patients and carers, who should be valued and included in care offered. Fourth, they advocate that interprofessional learning should be interactive and active, case-based or scenario-based. Finally, they advocate that interprofessional learning needs to take account of the students' level of development and be a thread throughout the course.

These sections have outlined the main themes that run through the literature and offer insight into the future needs for clinical placement experience. Having recognized these needs, the following sections outline three placement frameworks that have been used with speech and language therapy students on undergraduate and postgraduate qualifying courses, and discuss how the placements can address some of the issues highlighted. The placement formats are outlined in detail, considering them in the order they were first devised and implemented:

- mainstream school placement
- nursery placement
- acute hospital placement.

Mainstream school placement

Purpose and background

Paediatric speech and language therapy services have an increasingly large role to play in a school setting. Services to children in mainstream schools vary across the country, but the demand for the service usually outstrips the supply. The role of the therapist is most commonly that of collaboration/consultation. The child's communication abilities are assessed and the therapist gives advice to the class teacher or teaching assistant; if ongoing support for the child is available, the therapist leaves a programme and activities to be carried out until the next visit. Visits may be half-termly or termly.

The skills required of a qualified practitioner have therefore extended with this new consultative role. He or she is expected to have the skills of summarizing assessment results in a format accessible to teaching staff, and be able to interpret the results in the context of the client's need in an education setting. This requires knowledge of how the education setting operates and knowledge of classroom practice. It also requires negotiating skills and appreciation of another professional's role and pressures. Clinicians also need to have skills of therapeutic intervention with children, even though they will not be carrying out the programmes. In order to leave a suitable programme for a classroom assistant to carry out, they need to be able to predict how the child might respond, how quickly the programme might progress, what supports or cues the child might need, what sort of activities might be of interest and how to incorporate the programme into the curriculum. A student on placement with a busy therapist covering a number of mainstream schools may find it difficult to absorb all these skills, and may have little opportunity to work with a child on an ongoing basis. There may be limited opportunity for the student to talk to teaching staff, as the clinician will usually have far greater knowledge of the child under discussion, nor is there often time to spend in learning how the classroom functions. How might a placement be designed in order to offer the student a guaranteed opportunity for practising all these skills? What does the placement need to offer in order for students to develop the necessary skills to be fit for practice to work in schools?

Principles addressed by the placement

Many things were taken into consideration in the design of the new schools placement. First, from the literature outlined earlier, a main objective of the placement was to allow the students to develop some sense of themselves as a trainee practising professional. The placement was designed to encourage independent learning while maintaining support and supervision, encouraging the students to use staff as resources and recognizing when they needed guidance.

Second, the placement was designed to enable students to develop skills of working in an education setting and to give them time for liaison with teaching staff, learning to exchange information and work collaboratively in designing intervention programmes. Students would spend time in the classroom learning about the role of the teacher and pressures they are under. To reduce risk, but also to encourage collaborative working with peers, the students were placed in pairs in the schools, and given clients to work with, but it was left to the students to negotiate between them how they would arrange the sessions.

Third, to address the issue of experience alone not automatically leading to learning, the students were encouraged to keep reflective logs, which were handed in to a tutor each week. These proved to be an excellent way of keeping up with what the students were doing, and were used by the students to seek information, clarify their thinking and reflect on what they were doing.

The importance of students developing knowledge of evidence-based practice was addressed in sessions during the workshops. These were designed to give students the necessary skills to establish baseline measures and develop clear objectives for therapy which would be re-tested at the end of the block of intervention to give outcomes.

The placement was therefore designed to fulfil the aims of:

- developing theory in practice
- developing independent and interdependent learning
- increasing peer learning/teamworking skills
- developing interprofessional working, liaising with education staff

- promoting reflective learning
- providing a standardized experience
- increasing clinical skills of assessment and therapy
- increasing knowledge of an education setting and the place of communication skills in the curriculum
- developing knowledge of evidence-based practice.

Placement design

All students in the third year of the four-year undergraduate course undertook the placement. Students were paired up and assigned two children in a local school. The children were provided by the local service, and were children without statements who were known to the service but had no regular help in school. The requirements were that the clients should be non-complex, and that there should be potential for progress. The stipulation made to the schools was that there had to be a room available for the students to work in.

The placement model

Figure 6.1 outlines the placement model.

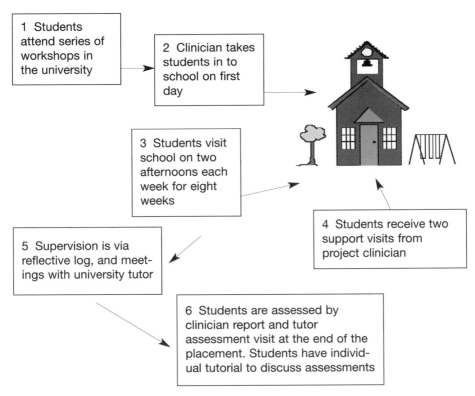

Figure 6.1 The mainstream school placement model.

Preparation for placement

The students received six half-day workshops prior to the placement, using the clients as case studies to discuss theory, preparing them for working in an education setting, covering issues of health and safety and behaviour management. A large proportion of the time was spent working with the case notes, giving students time to absorb all the information in them and to begin to make plans for further investigation or possible areas of intervention. This was done with support from tutors, and students were encouraged to begin to think about how to establish baselines, which could then be evaluated following the intervention. It was important to be mindful of the need to orientate the students to the learning experience, spending time outlining the learning principles that were being incorporated, explaining the approach and what the expectations were. During the workshops the students met the clinician whose child they would be seeing to discuss the case, and to arrange to meet at the school on the first day. Towards the end of the placement, the students were also required to prepare a short presentation on one of the children they had been working with in their pairs. The students gave the presentations in pairs, and they were watched by the other students, together with some members of staff. The students received feedback on their presentation skills, although it was not a formally assessed component of the placement.

Health and safety

Risk factors were reduced by the students working in pairs in a school with staff easily available, being made aware of health and safety requirements in the workshops, and checking and countersigning of case notes each week. The students could also seek advice from or raise concerns with their university tutors.

Outcomes

Students were asked to complete evaluation questionnaires following the placement, and these were compared with feedback from the standard placements offered to students the previous year. These questionnaires were designed for the project, however they have since been incorporated into routine placement evaluation of all placements on the course.

- 100% of students rated the placement as 'good' or 'excellent', compared with 84% of those who had traditional placements.
- 94% of students reported that they had gained 'a lot of insight' or 'excellent insight', compared with 63% who had traditional placements.
- 81% of students felt there had been 'good' or 'excellent' support, an almost identical pattern to the traditional placements.

The student feedback about the support received was extremely positive, as it offered a very different learning experience to being with a clinician. It was interesting therefore to see that the students' comments regarding the placement, via the feedback form, the reflective logs and discussion, were extremely positive, with the students reporting that they enjoyed the opportunity to learn independently. Typical comments were 'the placement allowed me to try things out for myself and learn by experience', 'it was an opportunity to build up confidence and realize that with practice and experience I would become a competent speech and language therapist', 'I will learn a lot from having to think for myself'.

- Students commented that they had been pleasantly surprised that they had been seen as colleagues by the teaching staff. Some of them found it amazing that they were listened to, as having information to impart to another professional.
- Students reported that they had found doing the presentations nerve-wracking, but had found it very helpful to hear about what other students were doing with their clients, and begin to explore similarities and differences. Tutors were initially surprised by this comment as it had been assumed – wrongly – that there had been discussion between students. It seemed that this was not the case, and in subsequent groups undertaking the placement there was specific effort to encourage the students to swap resources or ideas with other pairs, and even build up a resource bank for all to use.

From the university tutor perspective:

- The model provided a high number of standardized quality placements and there was no difficulty finding schools to participate. In feedback following the project they all wanted to participate again and would like increased numbers of students.
- The students all did well in their clinical assessments. When this group of students entered their final year, their reports from clinicians were positive. They reported that they had a good understanding of the educational setting and were independent learners. It will be interesting to look at the feedback forms from these students sought after a year in practice to see if their learning has indeed stood them in good stead for practice.
- The presentations, as well as giving the opportunity to swap ideas, were also useful in developing the skills of oral delivery of a case summary. Presentation of information to a group is a growing aspect of practising therapists' work, and an important skill to possess.
- The placement established a close working relationship between the university and the local service. The notion of a joint responsibility for providing training for the future workforce was a reality. Having a lead clinician within the local service during the project was extremely

valuable, and is a model similar to that of clinical teacher – a post jointly funded by a local service and a university to have a clinician in post with special responsibility and dedicated time for student training. Although common in medicine, this seems to be an underused model in speech and language therapy.

From the local clinicians perspective:

• The opportunity to supervise intensive intervention for children on their caseload proved to be extremely valuable. The project clinician called it 'an emptying of the guilt box', providing a service to those who haven't made progress through normal service delivery.
• Through the students setting clear baselines and measurable objectives with their clients, local clinicians developed skills themselves in this area.
• The project used students in a similar way to the way the service used assistants, but the clinicians were not required to provide the support and supervision, freeing up their time for other clients.
• The project was initially funded via confederation money, which paid the clinician and tutor for time to devise, implement and evaluate the initiative. The success of the project in terms of clinical placements (Baxter and Gray, 2001) and client outcome (Baxter and Merrils, 2001) has meant that the project has continued beyond the funding, and become incorporated into the local service's normal clinical placement provision. Clinicians are increasingly seeing students as a valuable resource.

Conclusions

The placement was developed in partnership with the local service and was extremely well received. It enabled students to gain valuable hands-on experience, and provided intervention to schoolchildren with high levels of need. The schools were extremely welcoming, valuing the student contribution highly. Students gained the opportunity to develop hands-on skills with clients that will stand them in good stead when they are enskilling others. They developed an understanding of a professional role, and of the education environment, developing independent learning strategies and the ability to work with others. The placement enables the university to provide a standardized experience for all students. The model has shown that by rethinking traditional models and looking at placement objectives more broadly, new methods of placement provision can be introduced successfully. By training providers and local services collaborating to develop new models, each can benefit.

Nursery placement

Purpose and background

This placement originated from work already in progress (Locke and Beech, 1991) looking at language levels of children in nursery schools within areas of high need. The study looked at language development as preparation for literacy, researching whether nursery teacher training in language work with children would boost impoverished language levels. A few students were originally recruited to work on the project as an addition to their clinical placements. They reported that they found the experience very worthwhile, so the possibility of extending it into a placement experience was pursued. As discussed in relation to the school project, the role of the speech and language therapist in education has increased considerably over the years, and there seem to be three main reasons for this. First, as therapists have become aware of the limitations of clinic-based work, they have looked to provide intervention in the child's communication environment. Second, as children have entered nursery education at a younger age, liaison with the education setting has needed to start earlier. And finally, as the importance of communication in the curriculum has been recognized, therapists have sought to integrate speech and language therapy into the child's school learning. Speech and language therapy graduates now need to enter the profession with the ability to work with colleagues from education, to assess children's communication levels, and plan joint goals and intervention. Hopefully, the days of therapists assessing children in clinic and posting a programme to a teacher have all but disappeared. Understanding each other's role, responsibilities and pressures is vital in order to provide effective client care.

As in the school placement, the main target was for students to develop the skills and knowledge that would enable them to be fit for practice in the field of education. The aim was for the students to begin to think of themselves as trainee professionals, and to be able to operate independently, although recognizing when they needed guidance. They would be working in an education setting, developing working relationships with teaching colleagues and learning to work together to assess and carry out intervention programmes. This placement was providing intervention to children who were not identified as having communication impairments, but impoverished language levels. In this aspect, students were learning to work within frameworks similar to government initiatives such as Sure Start, which aim to work with families from areas of high deprivation to provide support and intervention at an early stage. Speech and language therapy services are becoming increasingly involved with initiatives such as these, which increases the range of situations that graduates are expected to be able to operate within. The particular aims identified for this placement were similar to the school placement:

- develop skills of working interprofessionally with teachers
- incorporate theory in practice
- develop knowledge of nursery settings and communication in this context
- develop knowledge of relating communication goals to educational goals
- encourage independent and interdependent practice
- offer a standardized placement for the year group
- develop peer working skills
- develop skills of working with therapy groups
- develop evidence-based practice by establishing baselines and evaluating outcome
- reflect on practice.

Placement design

The placement was provided for students on the postgraduate course, in the final year of the two-year programme.

The placement model

The placement model is shown in Figure 6.2.

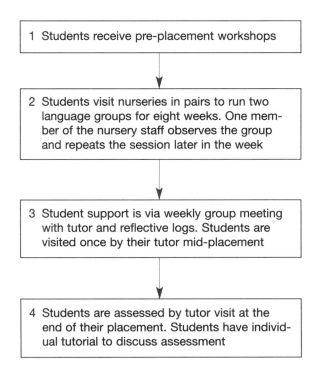

Figure 6.2 The nursery placement model.

Preparation for placement

The pre-placement workshops consisted of sessions including reminders of relevant theory, clinical methods, management of children, health and safety, sources of information and the important aspect of orientation to the learning, including how to work successfully with peers and what the expectations of the placement were. Following the placement, in addition to the individual feedback on the assessment, there was a group feedback and reflection session to swap experiences and discuss issues that arose.

Outcome

Student satisfaction with the placement, reported via placement feedback forms, has been high.

- Students have liked the independence and the chance to work in nurseries, feeling that they are colleagues and have a contribution to make.
- They have enjoyed the opportunity to work in groups, as much of their experience has been with individual therapy sessions, and the opportunity to work with children over a period of weeks to see change.
- They have also valued the opportunity to work on language rather than phonology, as much of their experience has been with children who have intelligibility difficulties, rather than working on skills of listening, understanding and using words and sentences in conversation.
- The reports from the nursery teachers have been extremely positive; they have found having the students working with them to be extremely valuable, and have appreciated the effort that the students have put into preparing the sessions and materials each week.
- Bearing in mind the feedback from the students on the school placement, a weekly informal meeting to swap ideas between students had been incorporated into the placement model, but this was received with a lack of enthusiasm, seeing it as extra time out of the week. It seemed that the students were happier swapping ideas informally with other students they knew, rather than having a formal session, and using the session instead as 'checking in' time for students needing advice.

From the university tutor perspective:

- It has been valuable to link the placement experience with ongoing research, to give the students the important message that research is not divorced from practice.
- The postgraduate students are particularly suitable for this type of independent placement experience as they enter the course with skills of adult learners.
- As with the school project, the placement provided a number of standardized, high-quality placements.
- The increasing emphasis on early years and preventative initiatives

requires graduating practitioners to be able to operate in new working environments; this placement encouraged students to consider these aspects.
- By working closely with nursery staff in planning sessions, students gained valuable insight into language in education and working with other professionals.

Discussion

This placement was originally developed from research data-gathering work, and reminds us of the close link between practice and research. The students enjoyed being part of the data gathering, and it was possible to use a different year group of students to gather data for the controls. Thus a second group of placements resulted from this project, providing valuable experience for those students in practising assessments and the establishment and re-evaluation of baselines. It is hoped in the future to link in with initiatives by local services to continue this pilot project in similar form. The funding for the support visits was provided by education action zone monies, which recognized the benefits to the nurseries and children involved. The demand for intervention in the early years of education and the numbers of children entering nursery with impoverished language levels, particularly in the inner cities, is huge. With a little creative thinking in placement design, the potential for students to gain valuable clinical experience while providing much-needed intervention programmes to this population need not be an untapped resource.

Acute hospital placement

Purpose and background

This placement was initially a means to alleviate a crisis in placement provision in the area of adult neurology, but has become a model of practice for promoting interprofessional working with patients following strokes. Finding sufficient placements for students in the area of adult neurology seems to have become increasingly difficult. There may be many reasons for this, including:

- the increasing proportion of working time that therapists spend with dysphagic clients, with whom students, having only done basic training, are not competent to work
- more senior staff are working with dysphagic clients, which leaves the junior staff to work with clients with communication difficulties. These junior staff may be too recently qualified to take students
- there are recruitment difficulties for more senior staff in the area of adult work.

These factors may contribute to a real difficulty in securing sufficient experience with adults for students. It is a worrying trend, as students who feel more confident working in paediatrics will tend to take jobs in this area, reducing the pool of future workers in the adult field, leading to less placement experience being provided.

This placement was developed, with funding provided by the local workforce confederation, to provide much-needed experience for students working with adults who have communication difficulties following strokes. It was offered at a local acute hospital and was designed to give students the opportunity to learn with, and from, students and professionals from other disciplines in client-centred workshops. The aims were to:

- give students experience of doing screening assessments on clients with communication difficulties following strokes
- develop understanding of other team members' roles with clients
- develop skills of exchanging information with professionals from other disciplines
- integrate theory and practice in case-based learning
- develop skills of joint care aim planning.

Design of placement

The placement was designed with a colleague from the local service, who is working in an acute hospital setting. The funding of the project via the workforce confederation paid for both clinician time and university tutor time to develop, carry out and evaluate the initiative. Students and professionals working within the hospital were invited along to the sessions, to observe the session and take part in the discussion that followed. There were at least two non-speech and language therapy participants at the sessions; they included physiotherapy students, occupational therapy students, nurse students, physiotherapists, occupational therapists or stroke nurses.

Placement model

1 In the clinic room, two speech and language therapy students carry out a screening assessment on a client with communication difficulties following a stroke (45 minutes). The clinician, other speech and language therapy students and the non-speech and language therapy participants monitor the proceedings from an observation room, via a one-way mirror and audio link.
2 The two students working with the client receive feedback from the clinician (15 minutes) and the observing group leave for a coffee break and informal discussion.
3 All participants meet in a larger discussion room, sitting in a semi-circle (1.5 hours).

4 The speech and language therapy participants explore the findings of the communication assessment under subheadings of areas of impairment. Each student in the group reports back on an area to the group, translating profession-specific terminology for other participants.
5 The non-speech and language therapy participants report back information about the patient from their professional perspective.
6 The participants discuss care aim priorities.
7 The two speech and language therapy students carrying out the session write up a care plan.

Outcome

All participants were asked to complete a feedback form following the sessions, with information in qualitative and quantitative form. Participants were asked what they had liked about the sessions and what they had not liked; they were also asked to respond to five questions about the sessions on a five-point 'strongly disagree' to 'strongly agree' scale.

All participants received the placement experience very positively.

- The most commonly quoted 'like' about the sessions by the speech and language therapy students was in relation to the discussion after the client had been seen. They had gained from the opportunity to apply their theory to the clients.
- The speech and language therapy students also reported satisfaction with the hands-on nature of the placement. As mentioned previously, placements with adult clients with neurological impairments are becoming increasingly difficult to find, particularly in acute hospital settings. Students had particularly appreciated the chance to try out and enhance hands-on skills, which will stand them in good stead for their further placements and exams. A particular strength of this model of placement provision was that it was experiential, not just observational.
- The speech and language therapy students had found the involvement of the other professions helpful, nine mentioning it specifically as something they had liked about the sessions. One student had a negative impression of this, however, feeling that it had reduced time available to discuss the communication aspects of the case. The non-speech and language therapy students had found the opportunity to learn about speech and language therapy assessment valuable, with little reported that had not been liked about the sessions.

From the university tutor perspective the sessions had been particularly valuable for the following reasons:

- They provided a standardized student placement experience, with the clinician able to prepare and select a range of clients for students to learn from.

- As the speech and language therapy students' knowledge and understanding of the communication abilities of the clients was at a deeper level than the qualified professionals and the students from the other professions, they had been forced to learn to 'decode' profession-specific knowledge and report their findings avoiding terminology. This enabled them to check and refine their own understanding, but also to practise clear communication, a vital skill for working with clients and other professionals.
- In clinical education, it is well recognized that it is not only the time spent with a client but the reflection and discussion following it that is of paramount importance. By discussion and interaction with clients, students were able to develop not only espoused theory but also theory in use. Students did not report that they felt that one client had been insufficient in a session, some felt that a longer session or even two sessions could have been devoted to a single client to give depth of learning. It is suggested that in-depth learning about a few clients can be preferable to students seeing a greater quantity of clients but with less discussion time.
- The students reported that a particularly valuable aspect of the placement was giving them the opportunity to discuss real clients and consider the theoretical considerations. This placement was designed to allow for in-depth discussion of clients, which is not often possible for clinicians in a busy clinic. By specifically paying attention to this discussion of theory, the students are developing their ability to use theory and make their own theory in use.

From the local service perspective, because clinician time is being paid for through the project funding, there is no constraint regarding small client numbers seen in these sessions. The attendance of qualified staff from the hospital has offered a useful opportunity for in-service training for these team members, and has given them valuable insight into communication difficulties in the clients they are working with. There is also the opportunity to use these sessions for staff development, for example returners to practice or newly qualified staff.

Discussion

The placement has been an excellent example of the university and local service working together to provide a learning opportunity, which would not otherwise have been available. At the first placement session, the speech and language therapy students were asked how many had talked to or observed a physiotherapist or occupational therapist working, or discussed an adult neurology case with another professional. Out of the group of 26, very few had ever had contact with another professional; where they had, it was usually through knowing another student or professional personally. It seems that many 'normal' placements provided in services are not able to provide this experience in addition to the hands-on practice with clients that students require. It would seem important that the method of working that is modelled to students by practising professionals is clearly that of working in interprofessional teams. If students are able to experience and see the benefits of this on placement, it will encourage them to adopt similar practices when they graduate. In addition to the placement feedback forms, the project has also gathered data regarding their views on interprofessional working and their attitude to interprofessional learning, which will be reported in the future.

As the sessions were led by speech and language therapists, there was inevitable bias towards this area. It would be interesting to extend this placement, with sessions being led in turn by professionals from different disciplines. As speech and language therapy accreditation requirements currently stand, however, sessions can only count towards professional practice hours if they are under the supervision of a qualified speech and language therapist. This clearly needs to be considered in the light of the drive towards interprofessional education.

Conclusions

The three placement models described in this chapter are examples of how rethinking a traditional model can yield benefits. By starting from the point of the learning objectives that the student needs to meet, rather than the placement experience offered, it is possible to consider change. The placements outlined here are offered to students as part of their training programme, and have been carefully planned into the curriculum to ensure that students are at the right level of ability to maximize their learning from them. Placements such as those described here are used in conjunction with other learning experiences, including the traditional one therapist to one student placement. This chapter has not argued that these traditional placements are obsolete, but rather that they offer the student particular learning experiences, which, as part of a package, provide valuable contributions. But the key seems to be that they are part of a package and combined with other experiences, which are able to achieve different objectives. Most student feedback is positive about traditional placements and it is important that this is not forgotten in a rush to introduce innovations. The principles of good clinical learning, such as the importance of students being given feedback on their performance and the need for clear learning objectives together with a transparent assessment process, are key aspects for traditional as well as new placement models.

The needs of practising professionals today seem to have expanded: there is now a requirement to be able to work in teams, to work collaboratively with other professionals and the client themselves, to have the ability to enskill others and to provide information in a clear, jargon-free way. The ability to manage caseloads, to provide outcome data, and to operate in a world of audit and clinical governance all provide challenges to the students who are graduating, to say nothing of the rapid changes in knowledge and information technology. In order to keep up to date, professionals are required to continue their professional development throughout their working lives; their training course before practice is now referred to in the literature as 'initial professional education', implying the ongoing nature of learning. It is important that students are encouraged to think in this way from their initial clinical placements, and to become active learners who can reflect on their own practice. What a challenge to educators to produce students who can cope with this demanding world.

The models presented in this chapter have gone a long way towards changing the impression that many practising clinicians have of students in training as being a burden that only take up their time. Instead, students are now being given credit for the skills and knowledge they possess, recognizing that they are not of course at the level required for practice. However, they can make useful contributions to the workforce, even during training, and providing they are given the necessary support and means to gain from experience, can operate as valuable 'free' labour. In the school project, clinicians thought of the students as speech and language therapy assistants, and because the support and supervision was being provided by the university and a project clinician, the students provided a valuable service in taking children off the clinicians' caseload for a while. Through joint placement design between local services and the university, it is possible to implement new models of placement, rather than just assuming that the way it has been done will always be the way it should be done. With the advent of health professional students receiving bursaries from the NHS, rather than student grants, the joint responsibility between training establishments and local services to train the future workforce has been brought sharply into focus. These placement models have shown that by universities and local services working together to design placements, high-quality student learning opportunities can be created.

Summary

This chapter has endeavoured to consider current literature relating to the area of clinical education and inform practice in the provision of clinical placements. It has considered assumptions that are made by the traditional form of placement and examined these assumptions with reference to available literature. It has then gone on to give examples of how rethinking the traditional model can offer new learning opportunities for students by services working in partnership with training establishments. At a time when training institutions are being asked to take more students onto their programmes to increase the workforce, and services are under intense pressure, the provision of adequate numbers of high-quality placements is becoming critical.

Clearly, decisions regarding the responsibility for the funding of clinical placements need to be considered. At present, placements are expected to be provided by clinicians working within the NHS, and there is little or no specific funding for speech and language therapy student workplace training. With the current shortage of clinicians in post and the pressures of maintaining client contacts, however, student placement considerations can often be considered a low priority by services. It has already been mentioned that the clinical teacher model, where clinicians are employed within services with special responsibility and dedicated time for student teaching, is an approach that could be utilized more fully. The models described in this chapter have all received funding in order to be devised and implemented, and can be maintained with relatively small amounts of funding, providing large amounts of student learning time cost-effectively.

Clinical education is becoming recognized as an area of learning in its own right, and there is an increasing literature to inform it, although considerably more remains to be done. However, there is a need for clinical education be recognized, to reward clinicians who excel in the area of teaching students, not just in clinical work, and to properly consider the provision of clinical placement experience in terms of content and quality rather than hours. In order to ensure that the students who are graduating are fit to practise in an ever-changing world, it is vital that their training prepares them adequately for this. Therefore the time for considering new models of clinical placements is here.

References

Argyris C, Schon D (1991) Participatory action research and action science compared: a commentary. In Whyte WF (ed.) Participatory Action Research. Newbury Park, CA: Sage.

Barr H (2000) Interprofessional Education: 1997–2000 A Review. London: UK Centre for the Advancement of Interprofessional Education.

Barr H, Freeth D, Hammick M, Koppel I, Reeves S (2000) Evaluations of Interprofessional Education: A United Kingdom Review for Health and Social Care. London: UK Centre for the Advancement of Interprofessional Education and British Educational Research Association.

Baxter S, Gray C (2001) The application of student-centred learning approaches to clinical education. International Journal of Language and Communication Disorders 36 (supplement): 396–400.

Baxter S, Merrils D (2001) Providing intensive therapy in schools for children with no identified provision. International Journal of Language and Communication Disorders 36 (supplement): 104–109.

Boud D (1988) Moving towards autonomy. In Boud D (ed) Developing Student Autonomy in Learning, 2nd edn. London: Kogan Page.

Boud D, Feletti G (1991) The Challenge of Problem-based Learning. London: Kogan Page.

Boud D, Keogh R, Walker D (1993) Using Experience for Learning. Buckingham: Society for Research into Higher Education and Open University Press.

Carr W, Kemmis S (1986) Becoming Critical: Education Knowledge and Action Research. Brighton: Falmer Press.

DoH (2000a) The NHS Plan: A Plan for Investments a Plan for Reform. London: Department of Health.

DoH (2000b) Meeting the Challenge: A Strategy for the Allied Health Professions. London: Department of Health.

Dreyfus H, Dreyfus S (1986) Mind Over Machine: The Power of Human Intuition and Expertise in the Era of the Computer. Oxford: Blackwell.

Eraut M (1994) Developing Professional Knowledge and Competence. London: Falmer Press.

Ewan C (1988) The social context of medical education. In Cox K, Ewan CE (eds) The Medical Teacher, 2nd edn. Edinburgh: Churchill Livingstone.

Finch J (2000) Interprofessional education and teamworking: a view from the education providers. British Medical Journal 321: 1138–1140.

Leathard A (1994) Going Interprofessional: Working Together for Health and Welfare. London: Routledge.

Lincoln M, Carmody D, Maloney D (1997a) Professional development of students and clinical educators. In McAllister L, Lincoln M, McCleod S, Maloney D (eds) Facilitating Learning in Clinical Settings. Cheltenham: Stanley Thornes.

Lincoln M, Stockhausen L, Maloney D (1997b) Learning processes in clinical education. In McAllister L, Lincoln M, McCleod S, Maloney D (eds) Facilitating Learning in Clinical Settings. Cheltenham: Stanley Thornes.

Locke A, Beech M (1991) Teaching Talking: A Screening Test and Intervention Programme for Children with Speech and Language Difficulties. Windsor: NFER-Nelson.

Lowry L, Burns C, Smith A, Jacobson H (2000) Compete or complement? An interdisciplinary approach to training health professionals. Nursing and Health Care Perspectives 21: 76–80.

Mezirow J (1983) A critical theory of adult learning and education. In Tight M (ed.) Adult Learning and Education: A Reader. London: Croom Helm and Open University Press.

Miller C, Freeman M, Ross N (2001) Interprofessional Practice in Health and Social Care: Challenging the Shared Learning Agenda. London: Arnold.

Morris C (2001) Student supervision: a risky business. International Journal of Language and Communication Disorders 36 (supplement): 156–161.

Parsell G, Bligh J (2001) Recent perspectives on clinical teaching. Medical Education 35: 409–414.

Schon D (1983) The Reflective Practitioner. London: Temple Smith.

Smith M, Barton J, Baxter J (1996) An innovative, interdisciplinary educational experience in field research. Nurse Educator 21: 27–30.

Stenglehoffen J (1993) Teaching Students in Clinical Settings. London: Chapman and Hall.

Taylor I (1997) Developing Learning in Professional Education: Partnership for Practice. Buckingham: The Society for Research into Higher Education and Open University Press.

PART III
INFORMATION TECHNOLOGY: DEVELOPMENTS AND APPLICATIONS

Chapter 7
Getting professional education online

MARGARET FREEMAN

Introduction

The last few years have seen major developments in the use of computers and networked technologies, in almost every aspect of daily life. In fact, the Internet, the World Wide Web and email have been described as 'transformational', because of their wide-ranging impact on the ways that people and organizations throughout the industrial world communicate and interact with each other (Salmon, 2000). This impact has certainly been felt throughout the education and healthcare sectors, as the possibilities for using networked communications in research, education and practice have been recognized and exploited for various aspects of our work (Pickering and McAllister, 1997; COT/CSP, 1999; Harden and Hart, 2002).

Like colleagues in other disciplines, health practitioners and those involved in pre-qualification professional education have recognized that we need to increase our understanding and use of computer-mediated technologies (Pickering and McAllister, 1997; Miller et al., 1997; Horton, 2001). However, it seems that action to adopt these technologies within the allied health professions has been generally slow and rather patchy, at least in the UK (COT/CSP, 2000; Hughes and Dewhurst, 2002). A survey of schools of therapy and professional bodies identified some of the reasons for this (Anthony, 2001). The majority of respondents stated that they had limited access to the appropriate resources, including the technical support and expertise to create and deliver online learning. In addition, these educators also questioned whether clinical learning, with its emphasis on interpersonal and interactive skills, could be delivered effectively in an online environment.

Despite this, some interesting and useful clinical applications of learning technologies have been designed and used for teaching in the therapies (Freeman et al., 1996; Lum and Cox, 1998; Oates and Russell, 1998; Boucher et al., 1999; Howard et al., 2001). The evaluations of these

145

and similar resources from cognate disciplines such as medicine (Bearman et al., 2001; Kneebone and ApSimon, 2001) show that well-designed computer simulations or video-based demonstrations can support effective and efficient learning for clinical practice. Indeed, it has been suggested that clinical simulations may be viewed as a 'marvellous medical education machine', which can overcome many of the problems of traditional clinical education (Friedman, 2000).

Of course, the role and functions of information and communication technologies (ICT) extend much further than these specific clinical applications. Like students in all other disciplines in the tertiary education sector, students in all professional disciplines should have opportunities to develop their understanding and use of ICT and networked learning as part of their general education (Dearing, 1997). Similarly, all students need to be equipped with the skills of information literacy and knowledge management, so that they can cope with the 'information explosion' which has been stimulated by web-based publishing in the past few years (Candy, 2000; McAvinia and Oliver, 2002). In professional courses, students also need to be equipped to respond to the increased use of ICT in all aspects of professional activity (Pickering and McAllister, 1997; COT/CSP, 2000; Grimson et al., 2000), especially in the UK health services, as the NHS Information Strategy becomes a reality (Milburn, 2001; DoH, 2001).

The recognition of the need for change is, of course, only the first step in the process of incorporating information technologies in our teaching and learning. It is widely acknowledged that the next stages, which involve making decisions about how to implement ICT – and then actually doing it – are the times when educators need the most support (Conole and Oliver, 1998; Bonk et al., 1999; McAvinia and Oliver, 2002). This includes opportunities to gain ideas about potential resources, to see them in action, to evaluate their usefulness and to gain advice about ways to adopt or adapt these resources to meet our own needs (Bonk et al., 1999; Anthony, 2001; Hughes and Dewhurst, 2002). The aim of this chapter is therefore to draw on the experiences of those who have already adopted information and learning technologies, in the hope that we can learn from examples of good practice and reflect on their relevance to pre-professional education.

Computer-mediated and networked technologies in teaching and learning

Ideas about the uses of ICT in education have evolved rapidly in the past ten years, partly as a result of technological development, but also because of the experiences gained in using the technologies. Even as the first generations of computer-assisted learning (CAL) resources were being evaluated (Timms et al., 1997), new opportunities were opened up by the capabilities of faster computers with multimedia facilities (Davies and Crowther, 1995). All of these developments were overtaken by the emergence of electronic networks. These have not only proved a major tool for educational delivery, but have also fostered global debate and research into the role of technology in the learning process, and about the processes of learning and teaching per se (Laurillard, 1993; Bonk et al., 1999; Phipps and Merisotis, 1999; Laurillard and McAndrew, 2002).

Although there is considerable overlap, we can identify several main themes in the literature about learning technologies, each of which has applications in clinical and professional education:

- learning and training courseware (or CAL), which is typically delivered as CD-ROMs or free-standing web-based study modules (Greenhalgh, 2001)
- computer simulations, including their uses for clinical training
- accessing and using the World Wide Web as an information resource and the implications for information literacy and knowledge management
- using networked learning in the curriculum
- informal e-learning, often used in workplace learning or continuing professional development, to support communication via web pages, video-conferencing and email discussion groups.

CAL and other learning and training resources

Computer assisted learning packages are perhaps the most well-known form of learning technology. They are often presented in CD-ROM format and use multimedia combinations of sound, graphics, text and moving images to present information and tasks in an attractive and user-friendly way (Vogel and Wood, 2002). CAL approaches have been used to promote self-help and self-study for a wide range of purposes.

Because they have a comparatively long history and have been used so widely, the experiences of using CAL resources provide useful insights into the benefits and limitations of using these – and to some extent, other – forms of computer technology.

One of the most obvious uses of CAL is to facilitate 'deliberate practice' (Ericsson et al., 1993), which can be defined as:

> repetitive performance of intended cognitive or psychomotor skills in a focused domain, joined by rigorous skills assessment that provides the learners with specific, informative feedback, that results in increasingly better skills performance, in a controlled setting. (Issenberg et al., 2001)

Although this type of 'training' function has sometimes been assigned low status by some educators (Drew, 1998; McAvinia and Oliver, 2002), the mastery of most core skills and basic knowledge requires opportunities to build up levels of competency through repeated practice (Treadwell et al., 2002). As Schön (1987) pointed out, just as learning to play scales and arpeggios is a prerequisite for skilled performance with a musical instrument, the mastery of basic skills and knowledge provides the foundation stones of reflective professional practice. Multimedia packages have been shown to be effective and efficient for promoting skill-based learning. This is particularly the case when the packages offer graded learning activities, presented with interesting graphics and interactive exercises, with the opportunities for repeated practice and feedback on performance. The European Computer Driving Licence, which aims to promote basic computer competencies through self-study supported by intermittent class contact, is one example of this type of approach. The 'packaged' materials available for teaching and therapy (such as Earobics, Widgit software and SpeechViewer used in speech and language therapy), which use video game formats to promote basic skills are other examples of this type of application.

In tertiary education, CAL is typically used to complement and extend the learning opportunities provided by other modes of teaching (Davies and Crowther, 1995; Hughes and Dewhurst, 2002). The aim is to enable learners to build up their understanding and/or skills in 'a rich environment for active learning' (Grabinger and Dunlap, 2000). According to Vogel and Wood (2002: 214) multimedia and CAL have 'several advantages over paper and the spoken word, namely interactivity, the immediacy of graphics and the moving image, instantaneous navigation and searchability'. This makes them particularly useful for subjects which are 'visually intensive, detail oriented and difficult to conceptualise' (Greenhalgh, 2001: 42) such as biomedical science topics (Issenberg et al., 2001; Hughes and Dewhurst, 2002; Steele et al., 2002). According to Issenberg et al. (2001), there are now hundreds of CD-ROM programs available for learners at all levels, which teach anatomy and physiology, radiology, advanced cardiac life support, skills and procedures, and physical diagnostic techniques.

Promoting effective use of CAL

Although there are indications that well-designed CAL packages can promote deep, retentive learning (Vogel and Wood, 2002), there is also strong evidence that the way these packages are introduced and used can strongly influence their effectiveness (Davies and Crowther, 1995; Timms et al., 1997; Greenhalgh, 2001; Hughes and Dewhurst, 2002). Greenhalgh (2001) states that recognized barriers include inadequate planning, poor integration with other forms of learning and cultural resistance of staff. Hughes and Dewhurst (2002) add that educators need to provide time and support if students are to accept and use the resources appropriately. This includes making sure that the students are comfortable with computer technology in general, which means we need to provide them with opportunities to become familiar with the specific 'mechanics' of any new program before they are expected to use it for independent computer-based learning (Salmon, 2000). This has been emphasized in a number of studies: the evidence is mounting that students who lack confidence and competence with ICT are at a disadvantage when using CAL programs (Russell, 1995; Watson, 2001).

Computer simulations for professional teaching and learning

Educators in many healthcare disciplines have recognized that multimedia technology offers new possibilities for teaching and learning. Although the designs vary, there is strong emphasis on the use of experiential learning, through simulations or videos of real patients. Typically, the objective is to promote clinical reasoning and clinical skills, prior to the students' contact with 'real' clients (Christie et al., 2000).

Although the design and development of computer simulations tends to require a considerable amount of time and expertise (Koller, 2000), this can be balanced against the practical and educational benefits for the teachers, learners and patients. Henderson (1998), for example, observes that multimedia overcomes many of the practical constraints of a real-life clinic, while enabling the educator to design learning activities to match the needs of the students. An additional advantage is that 'virtual' patients are always available, which means that the programme of clinical learning activities can be planned with the certain knowledge that all students have equal opportunities for observation and interaction with appropriate clients, in a specific time frame (Bryce et al., 1998; Lum and Cox, 1998). Several educators have also noted that the time span can be optimized in virtual tutorials. Watson (2001) reports that students can work through up to 12 computer simulations in one hour, whereas in the 'real' laboratory, one of these experiments may take up to six weeks. In a similar vein, Bryce et al. (1998) note that students can obtain a more comprehensive picture of the diagnostic work-up of a patient when the real-time waiting for laboratory and other investigations is removed by the use of virtual tutorials.

Students value simulations because they provide working examples of clients' problems, with opportunities to learn how to carry out tests and procedures without fear of upsetting the client. Multimedia simulations also allow students to pause to check information, or to discuss their findings while working through the problem, and return to the same unchanging patient as often as they wish, in their own time, and to practise their skills at their own pace (Bryce et al., 1998). This means that 'real' patients benefit, because the students have already mastered the procedural aspects of the tasks being undertaken and thus are more able to give their attention to their interaction with the client.

The uses of computer simulations and virtual tutorials

The designs of virtual simulations tend to fall into two broad categories: those based on a problem-solving approach (DxR Development Group, 2001; DxRNursing, 2002; Nursing; Lum and Cox, 1998) and those which use a tutorial, or guided learning approach, often based on a specific topic (Freeman et al., 1996; Henderson, 1998). Although there are differences in the way the materials are presented and used, all of the tutorials aim to engage the student in active learning through case studies or clinical scenarios, with tutorial guidance and feedback. All of them also provide opportunities for learning about practice in the context of 'a virtual world, relatively free from the pressures, distractions and risks of the real one, to which, nevertheless, it refers' (Schön, 1987).

The problem-solving approach

DxR (2001), DxR Nursing (2002) and PATSy (PATSy, 2003) are examples of this type of learning resource. Essentially, they are databases for case studies of patients, each with a detailed case history and comprehensive battery of assessments. The task for the student is to gather the appropriate data in order to make a diagnosis and, in some cases, to plan the appropriate care. The value of this type of learning resource is that it provides students with opportunities to learn by doing, as they undertake assessments (Lum and Cox, 1998) and develop clinical understanding and reasoning through the process of synthesizing and integrating the information.

From their experience of using this approach with medical students, Bryce et al. (1998) report that it allows students to work through a realistic clinical situation, in which the patient may present with minimal information ('I have a pain in my chest') after which the data gathering is dependent on the clinician's actions in obtaining information from the patient, defining the problem, undertaking tests and interpreting the results. Unlike a 'real' clinic, where they rarely see one patient through a complete diagnostic regime, the simulation provided by DxR provides the opportunity to explore all aspects of each case in detail, to see the results of all tests and procedures, and to obtain feedback throughout. The PATSy system offers an additional benefit because most of the data are stored as short digitized video clips of patients with communication impairments, which also enables students to develop skills such as observation, test administration and interpretation of test results (Lum and Cox, 1998). The opportunity to elaborate their knowledge of communication impairments (Coles and Holm, 1993) through comparisons of data from different clients is also possible (see Chapter 8 for more details).

Virtual tutorials and guided learning with simulations

Whereas the designs described above aim to promote active learning through problem solving, other types of design have a number of similarities with what Wang and Bonk (2001) describe as 'electronic cognitive apprenticeship'. These authors suggest that this 'draws its inspiration from traditional apprenticeship and creates a meaningful social context in which learners are given many opportunities to observe and learn expert practices ... [by] ... solving real world problems under expert guidance that fosters cognitive and meta-cognitive skills and processes' (Wang and Bonk, 2001: 132).

All of the tutorials described below have been designed to support the development of the domain-specific skills which are essential components of professional competence. Thus, the designs include the overt guidance of an expert practitioner/clinical educator and the use of 'instructional methods' such as modelling, coaching, scaffolding, articulation, reflection and exploration (Collins et al., 1989) and/or questioning, task structuring, performance feedback or management, and direct instruction where appropriate (Wang and Bonk, 2001). In their model of cognitive apprenticeship, Wang and Bonk (2001) suggest that these instructional methods are effective when combined with real-life problems, learner involvement, and active application of knowledge and skills.

Teaching domain-specific skills

Although the need to achieve appropriate levels of expertise is emphasized in education for all professions, in reality the opportunities for developing these skills can be limited, as Kneebone and ApSimon (2001) highlight in their discussion of surgical skills. Despite the pre-qualification opportunities for knowledge acquisition and deliberate rehearsal of the basic techniques, these authors note that practice with simulated tissue 'in isolated skills workshops' without 'the cognitive context' does not provide the appropriate conditions required to master and maintain these skills at appropriate level.

Their solution has therefore been to develop a programme of 'focused practice within a framework of structured information to develop surgical skills' (Kneebone and ApSimon, 2001: 911). This framework includes a CD-ROM which 'presents the key components of a skill by progressing logically from explanation (using animation) to clinical demonstration (using video) to technical demonstration (on a model), thereby paving the way for supervised practice'. The CD-ROM is used by an expert surgeon-tutor, who 'talks through' the procedures with small groups (around 24 trainees) prior to more intensive one-to-one supervision and training. At the request of the trainees, Kneebone and ApSimon have made the CD-ROM available for further independent study and rehearsal.

Although the example of surgery per se is not directly relevant to students in the allied health professions, this model of providing opportunities for a variety of managed learning experiences can readily translate into other clinical scenarios. Howard et al. (2001), for example, have developed an integrated, multidisciplinary multimedia CD-ROM package (ViSuAL CLIP) for student speech and language therapists. The tutorial, based on digitized video and audio data from a four-and-a-half-year-old girl with specific language impairment, offers students the opportunity to analyse the data from different disciplinary perspectives, including linguistics, phonetics, speech and language pathology, and clinical management, each at different levels of complexity. The tutorial is designed with modular architecture, so that each module is free-standing, but can be linked to others. The modules are grouped into three sections:

- observation (including observation of assessment procedures for language and speech)
- teaching modules, which enable the student to engage in deliberate practice of phonetic transcription and to compare their results with those of the tutor
- reference modules, which provide extensive background material, including case history material, bibliographic references, normative data for speech and language acquisition, and relevant guidance notes for phonetic and phonological description.

Like Kneebone and ApSimon (2001), Howard et al. (2001) aim to ensure that the guided experiential learning enables the students to deepen their understanding and strengthen the skills already learned, in an applied clinical context. Oates and Russell (1998) have used a similar approach to promote the skills of perceptual analysis of clients with voice disorder and to link these to the physiology of the larynx. This package presents a number of clients with different degrees of vocal impairment, using video-recorded interview, case history and endoscopic data, acoustic data and animations of the larynx. The students undertake evaluations of each client, and these can be compared with the findings of a panel of expert clinicians for feedback.

Interviewing and communication skills

Although teaching communication skills via a computer may sound like a contradiction, a small number of studies have demonstrated that interactive tutorials can be used effectively to raise awareness and use of appropriate questioning styles (Bearman et al., 2001) to increase the skills of interpreting and responding to non-verbal communication and to promote the skills required for interviewing (Hulsman et al., 1999, 2002; Liaw et al., 2000).

In a slightly different context, Freeman et al. (1996) developed a tutorial based on a real-time interview with a real-life patient with a voice disorder. Like others, these clinical educators had used both video and expert demonstrations of the initial diagnostic interview, but had recognized that both of these methods had limitations. A particular concern was that both of these presentation modes place a heavy demand on students' cognitive processing, especially when a complex interaction is observed in real time. As well as the demand on memory and recall, it was recognized that novice observers can feel unsure of their understanding and doubt their ability to judge the salience of the information gained during these observations. The aim was therefore to provide tutorial guidance, commentary and questions for students as they worked through one example of an interview, so that the process and content were made explicit.

The tutorial, written by the expert therapist and the course tutor, is interwoven with the full 45-minute video-recorded interview and preliminary assessment. The digitized video pauses at intervals so that tutorial questions, commentary or other signposts for learning can mark significant events; model answers and further commentary are also provided. A recent revision of the tutorial (Freeman, 2001) includes hotlinks to relevant websites and additional commentary to emphasize the theoretical issues raised in the interview.

Used within the formal teaching programme, the tutorial allows all students to engage in active learning, to test and develop their understanding of both theory and process, and to undertake some rating or scoring of assessment results. The data from the case history are then used in class to discuss care planning (Malcomess, 2001) and therapy approaches, using the specific case as an exemplar. Also, students who are assigned to clinical placements in voice clinics can elect to revisit the tutorial to rehearse the domain-specific skills of interviewing, demonstration and explanation.

The virtual practicum

Henderson's (1998) virtual practicum centres on the diagnosis and long-term management of a simulated patient attending the virtual HIV/AIDS clinic and is intended for use by the multidisciplinary team. The whole tutorial is constructed as a series of rooms, which give access to the interviews, tests and treatment that occurred during the various stages of the patient's story. Interviews with actual patients, mini-lectures, case discussions with master clinicians and problem-solving activities are also included. Although this was a major project that required extensive time and funding, Henderson (1998) asserts that it demonstrated that simulation offers the necessary conditions for effective and efficient learning, which 'can at least supplement, and perhaps greatly improve on, real-life clinical education'.

Evaluations of simulations and multimedia learning resources

The evaluations of multimedia simulations have demonstrated that they can be effective and powerful learning tools which provide valid opportunities for experiential learning (Liaw et al., 2000; Issenberg et al., 2001). The simulations are valued by the students because they make explicit links between campus-based and work-based learning, enabling them to develop their understanding and use of theory-in-action at their own pace (Schön, 1987), and to develop some of the cognitive, motor and perceptual skills in preparation for work with 'real' clients.

There is no doubt that virtual tutorials are relatively expensive to produce, in terms of the time and expertise required for the design and production. However, these costs are at least partially offset by the fact that the resources are reusable and provide equal opportunities for experiential learning for large numbers of students. They also provide a controlled, student-centred learning experience, which overcomes some of the problems associated with live clinical experience, where access to appropriate clients is not guaranteed and the time available for learning tends to be limited by the service demands (Friedman, 2000; Ziv et al., 2000). According to Issenberg et al. (2001: 21) 'simulations and virtual reality hold out the promise of unlimited access to deliberate practice as part of skills training. As the skills required for practice ... become more numerous and more complex, such access to practice and rehearsal will become more essential.'

Accessing the Web and promoting information literacy

The two functions of the World Wide Web

The World Wide Web can be viewed as having two main functions in education: information provision and education provision (Bonk et al., 1999). Its first, general, function as an information provider, offers opportunities for almost everything from promoting products (which includes information about departmental and institutional achievements) to discovery learning (Laurillard, 1993) about almost any subject, from different perspectives and with different levels of complexity (Tait 1997).

Bonk et al. (1999) state that the Web offers almost endless opportunities for teaching, but they also suggest that it is possible to start using it as an information provider, with only minor adaptations to one's teaching. They outline a ten-level continuum of integration for Web-based learning, which begins with promoting the Web as an information resource and moves gradually to using it to develop different types of learning activities. This type of approach has a number of advantages, because it not only starts with the networking resources which are already available within the higher education institute, but also helps to raise awareness about the value and importance of computer technology in both the educational and working/experiential context.

Decisions about how far to progress with Web-based teaching will depend on the resources available and the 'comfort level' of the teachers and the students. It can also be argued, however, that educators need to move out of their 'comfort zone', if they are to optimize their own and their students' use of electronic resources (McVay Lynch, 2002)

Enabling students to use computers and networked resources

Koschman (1995) suggests that most of us go through three phases in our use of computer technology: *learning about computers*, as a precursor to *learning through computers* (i.e. using computers as tools for study and coursework) and *learning with computers*, as part of the day-to-day learning process. Although most of our students now enter higher educataion with basic competencies in ICT (the first of Koschman's phases), the evidence from various sources indicates that they still tend to require support to use the technology effectively for independent learning (OFSTED, 2002).

Even if only the most basic Web access is available, it is essential that all students in higher education can access and use electronic resources competently, if they are to make the transition to learning through and with the Internet and the Web. According to Reingold (1995): 'Fear is an important element in every novice computer user's first attempts to use a new machine or new software; fear of destroying data, fear of hurting the machine, fear of seeming stupid in comparison to others, or even to the machine itself'. There is strong evidence that fear or lack of familiarity with the technology can limit students' conceptual gains when using learning technology, whereas students who use the Web regularly seem to be able to adapt to using other new technologies (Watson, 2001).

Three factors tend to facilitate the transition from computer illiteracy to computer competence. The first is that the technology is available – which certainly should be the case in higher education institutes (Dearing, 1997). The second is that it is used and accepted within the educational culture, for coursework, general communication and information sharing (Bonk et al., 1999; Hughes and Dewhurst, 2002). The third is that time, support and opportunities to become familiar with the institution's procedures, such as logging on, sending and receiving emails, and navigating networks, are provided as part of the general induction to the degree course or in a study skills module (Bonk et al., 1999; McAvinia and Oliver, 2002).

Using the Web as an information resource

According to Bonk et al. (1999), the first phase of using the Web as an information resource begins with the general type of information about the department, the course and course modules which is usually made available via publicly accessible websites to prospective and current students, in most higher education institutes. The departmental website can also include a section with hotlinks to recommended websites. This step, of course, still requires that teacher or technician skills to convert documents into HTML format are available. However, the effort is worthwhile if the relatively low demands on the educator are viewed as a way of setting the students on the path towards exploring 'the vast stores of knowledge in which a field is based' (Bonk et al., 1999: 2). As the competencies and confidence of staff and students increase, decisions about further use of Web-based learning can be made.

Establishing competence and confidence with ICT

There is no doubt that induction and guidance from an enthusiastic and sympathetic educator or other experienced person is essential when any new form of electronic media is introduced (Draper et al., 1994). Therefore, even a brief introductory session to provide hands-on experience of logging on and undertaking small navigation tasks can be useful as part of the induction programme for new groups of students. Identifying the students who are computer confident and pairing them with their less confident peers is a useful strategy, so that peer support can be encouraged and established as part of the learning process.

In our own experience, introductory sessions run collaboratively by a course tutor and subject liaison librarian have proved a useful way of providing basic support for the 'mechanics' of the network, while also encouraging the students to consider the relevance of ICT for their current learning and future professional activity. This is provided via a 'hands-on' session in a computer suite, where students are first encouraged to log on and become familiar with procedures such as using their university network passwords. Following this, they are encouraged to locate key sites, including the departmental website, library pages, reading lists and the library catalogue (in accordance with Bonk et al.'s (1999) recommendations above).

The brief introduction is followed by an introduction to a general Web search engine (such as Google) on any topic relating to speech and language therapy. Because the students are encouraged to ask questions as they search, discussions arise about various issues, from how to copy, paste, store and print information, to questions about the differences between popular general search engines and specialist databases. This exercise also allows helps to encourage the use of effective strategies for the choice of search terms. For example, using a broad search term such as 'speech and language' produces almost two million citations from Google, which clearly demonstrates the need to narrow the search field. This session also provides the opportunity to guide students to the uses of other, perhaps more appropriate sources of information, such as the texts, journals and electronic sources identified on the course reading lists.

Encouraging students to email useful information to the study group's email list at this stage ensures that they have mastered skills such as using attachments and, if nothing else, should be more able to communicate with each other and respond to departmental email bulletins. This can be taken a step further, however, if resources are available to collate all the information in a course website or bulletin board, so that all students can see the value of pooling resources – Stage 2 on the continuum described by Bonk et al. (above).

Reinforcing learning through use

As with all new skills, it is important that the learning is maintained and extended by further use. The example above is reinforced by the tutor, who emails the group after the session to ask for feedback and also to encourage them to reply with a summary of their learning from the session. The problems identified within the group of students are then addressed in the next session of the study skills and professional learning module. Students are also encouraged to visit some of the introductory websites for computer-related skills (Cooper, 2002; NMAP, 2002) to check out their understanding and competency. Occasional problem-solving sessions, scheduled by the tutor and/or a supportive computer technician help to reduce anxieties and provide opportunities for trouble shooting. Although these sessions may become redundant, because members of the student group quickly begin to pool their expertise, it still remains important to provide time for orientation for any new type of computer-mediated learning program (Draper et al., 1994).

Developing information skills

As students progress through the course, they should be offered opportunities to extend their ICT and generic learning skills. Building in formal times to revisit these skills throughout the course can, according to McAvinia and Oliver (2002), enable students to reflect on their learning needs in terms of 'changes in ability and the identification of the next areas for learning ... [which] ... sets in motion the habits that will enable a student to become a lifelong learner (cf. Kolb, 1984)'.

When they are led by the specialist subject/liaison librarian, these sessions encourage awareness and use of relevant resources. Speech and language therapy students, for example, need to know how to access and use databases for a wide range of subjects and, as each of the database systems operates differently, it is useful to ensure that students are aware of these and can use appropriate search procedures. However, all clinical students should be introduced to concepts of medical informatics so that they can access the increasingly vast range of sources of medical and health-related information sources (Brandt et al., 1996; Hasman, 1998; Grimson et al., 2000; Staggers et al., 2000) through their own targeted searches and the use of specific healthcare sites and subject gateways (NELH, 2002; NMAP, 2002). Similarly, an introduction to the core information systems used in the NHS should be included, especially as the NHSNet is becoming more widely used in clinical practice (COT/CSP, 2000).

Students value the opportunity to review and replenish their information skills at different stages in the course. As well as the obvious need to include search skills and referencing systems as part of research design and methodology courses, in the later stages of the course they should be familiar with professional resources. In the context of speech and language therapy, for example, this includes the RCSLT (RCSLT, 2002) and American Speech-Language-Hearing Association (ASHA, 2002) websites, sites maintained by individuals (Bowen, 2002; Kuster, 2002) and organizations (RNID, 2002; MENCAP, 2002). The value of email, mailing and discussion lists in supporting continuing professional development through informal learning may also be addressed in these sessions (Allan, 2002).

Evaluating accuracy of websites

Pickering and McAllister (1997: 275) have observed that educators in the healthcare professions have an obligation to enable students to 'make critical judgements about the authority of information' available on the Web. As the next sections suggest, this not only has implications for the students' 'academic' learning, but can also have direct implications for professional practice.

Many websites now provide support for direct work with patients and carers, including ideas and examples of therapy materials and techniques (Wilson, 2001; Bowen, 2002; Hooper, 2002; Kuster, 2002) or information and advice literature for carers (ASHA, 2002; MENCAP, 2002; NINDS, 2002; RCSLT, 2002; RNID, 2002). While most of these sites, especially those produced by informed professionals and organizations, contain excellent information, wide variations have been identified in the quality of the information available on the Internet (Grimson et al., 2000; Gagliardi and Jadad, 2002; Purcell et al., 2002).

Students therefore need to know how to evaluate the accuracy, completeness and consistency of the material they access for their own use (Pickering and McAllister, 1997) and in preparation for potential discussions with clients and their carers (Roberts and Copeland, 2001; Purcell et al., 2002). This should include consideration of good and poor practice and codes of conduct in web design, including indications such as the identification of the author of the web page, acknowledgements of organizational (for example commercial) affiliations, indications of when the material was last updated, use of references, and the appropriateness of the language and content of the website (Bader and Braude, 1998; Kunst et al., 2002).

Citing sources and combating plagiarism

One of the downsides of the increased use of the Web is that plagiarism has become increasingly common. Because the facilities for cutting and pasting are readily available, students (and others) can easily 'lift' information from a Web-based source and, either accidentally or deliberately, insert it into their own work – and even into their websites (Anonymous, 2001; Stubley, 2002). As well as emphasizing the reasons to avoid, and the consequences of, plagiarism, all educators and librarians need to ensure that good practice in using and recording referenced material and citations is engrained into students' learning behaviours and demonstrated in all our own work. A comprehensive guide to good practice is available on the Joint Information Systems Committee website (JISC, 2002). The conventions for citing websites as references in academic writing (JISC, 2002), as well as the need for recording all sources of information used in any form of study, should be emphasized routinely.

Clients and patients as information seekers

Users of healthcare services make up one of the largest groups searching the Web for information (Ball and Lillis, 2001; Wilson, 2002). If they have the time and expertise, patients and their carers can access the full range of electronic resources, from personal accounts and user discussion groups to peer-reviewed articles and clinical decision support tools, before they seek a professional consultation. There are certainly anecdotal reports of patients having more current information than their doctor or healthcare worker (Grimson et al., 2000; Purcell et al., 2002) and of doctors telling their patients 'Whatever you do, don't go on the Internet' (Ferguson, 2002a: 555).

Ferguson's view is that accurate information can empower patients and their carers if it enables them to take an active part in the decision-making process about treatment options and management strategies. Ball and Lillis (2001) also point out that good consumer information is essential for disease prevention and management, as well as for the promotion of wellbeing. In support of this, Ferguson (2002b) has published guidelines on the Web to support effective information seeking by patients, which can also be of use to students and healthcare workers. As Leydon et al. (2000) point out, however, we also need to recognize the need for sensitivity about the timing and amount of information provided, because patients' information needs may vary at different times during any illness or episode of healthcare.

Using networked learning technologies in the curriculum

To a degree, some of the activities described above can be incorporated into an existing course without too much additional work on the part of educators or the students. It could be argued, for example, that enabling students to use the Web effectively and efficiently for independent study may save them time, as well as extending their use of resources. From a purely practical viewpoint, however, it is apparent that we cannot expect to keep adding extra elements into a curriculum that is already demanding. In addition, there is strong evidence that students do not use electronic resources optimally (if at all) when they are an optional extra. Students are more motivated to use the resources if they are perceived as an integral and relevant part of the course and/or the use of the resources contributes to assessment (Hughes and Dewhurst, 2002).

Integrating Web-based learning

One of the most obvious ways to promote integration of Web-based learning into the course is to reallocate some of the time from the face-to-face teaching programme so that the students can use relevant electronic resources, with the educator available for tutorial guidance and support. Alternatively, students could be assigned a case from a database (e.g. PATSy) to discuss in a tutorial.

One excellent example of an assignment which demonstrates the value of making the Web relevant for students is Celia Hooper's (Hooper, 2002) course website. This has been regularly updated with information on a wide range of topics related to the subject (voice disorder and voice therapy). The website is managed by Hooper, but contains a substantial section for information researched by the students as part of their coursework. By mounting this resource on a site that has open access, Hooper enables the students to see the value of their own work and to gain from the contributions of their peers. These students, and others, can also continue to use the site in the future to update their knowledge for continuing professional development. Hooper has ensured that students recognize the value of their contributions by: (a) inviting visitors to the site to send feedback by email; and (b) publicizing the site via the SID3 Voice email discussion forum. This type of approach is very similar to some of the suggested activities in Bonk et al.'s (1999) ten-stage continuum.

Virtual learning environments

Sometimes described as 'a course in box' (Anthony, 2001), virtual learning environments (VLEs) such as Blackboard, WebCT or First Class have been adopted by many higher education institutes. Essentially, a VLE is a package of integrated Web-mounted 'tools', which can be used to support online study through distance learning or campus-based teaching (O'Leary, 2002). The tools can be used quite flexibly to provide course support materials such as handouts, supplementary materials, graphics, links to other Web resources, and digitized video and audio-recordings. They also provide bulletin boards for asynchronous discussions and live chat rooms. The RCSLT website provides a useful demonstration of some of these features, which are being used by an increasing number of clinicians and students for information sharing and informal continuing professional development activities.

As a learning resource, VLEs can support a wide range of different approaches to teaching and learning. They could, for example, be used with first-year students to present fairly didactic, teacher-led complements to conventional face-to-face teaching, with the email tool providing individual students with the chance to contact the course leader with specific individual queries. As the degree course progresses and the students (and educators) become more familiar with the VLE tools, the amount of student-led activity may be increased. This may begin with encouraging the students to use the bulletin board facility for small group tutorial discussions of topics suggested by the tutor or to solve problems and answer queries raised by the students.

Because students can leave and read messages on the bulletin board at any time, this can be used between formal periods of class contact. The use of the bulletin board, and indeed any form of electronic discussion, tends to take some time to establish and needs quite a lot of support and encouragement from the discussion leader (Duggleby, 2000; Salmon, 2000). This may change, of course, because at least a proportion of students already have experience of socializing in chat rooms. However, it is recognized that students respond to both synchronous (chat) and asynchronous (bulletin board) tutorials in different ways. As in any other tutorial discussion, some students tend to take a more passive ('lurking') role in the discussions. Others may prefer asynchronous discussions to face-to-face tutorials because they have time to reflect and consider as they write a contribution to a bulletin board. The written transcript on the bulletin board also provides a record of the tutorial discussion, to which students can return for further reflection.

As more NHS clinics are provided with network connections, students should be able to access the course resources in the VLE which are relevant to their current clinical population. They could also use the chat room and bulletin board for discussions of current cases and clinical issues among themselves and/or between students and tutors, which could help to strengthen the links between the clinical and the campus-based components of the course.

A further possibility, if student-led discussion can be supported and developed through ongoing experience of using networked discussion, is that it may eventually be feasible to use computer-mediated communication (Salmon, 2000) as the main mode of learning and teaching in the latter stages of the degree course. This would enable the students to develop their concepts of collaborative and independent learning, as well as supporting a more flexible programme of study. If this were planned as a natural extension of their previous use of networked learning, it could also be a useful transition to their use of the Web for continuing professional development. The literature on networked learning (Bonk et al. 1999; McConnell, 2000; Salmon, 2000; McAteer and Harris, 2002; McVay Lynch, 2002) is replete with discussions about how to carry this forward.

Informal learning and continuing professional development

The electronic network has the potential to support continuing professional development by linking clinicians who have common areas of specialism via email, professional discussion groups and online conferencing. In fact, some UK professionals are beginning to use various discussion forums to share ideas and information. Over 150 people have joined the RCSLT bulletin board (The Coffee Shop) since it opened in late 2001, with contributions ranging from clinical queries to information about employment and pay scales. The number of email discussion lists has also increased in the last year; each has a sizeable membership and, in some cases, very active and lively discussions of topical issues.

This indicates that at least some members of each profession are already able to use e-communications for informal, workplace learning and raises interesting possibilities for future developments. One obvious example is that the activities of special interest groups and specialist advisors could be extended by the use of discussion lists. The potential for using more online conferencing for formal activities to support continuing professional development has already been recognized by some universities, such as the University of Greenwich, which offers an online, part-time MSc course in Continuing Professional Development (Health). Similar developments, including modular programmes for continuing professional development are planned by the NHS University (DoH, 2002)

Conclusion

It is apparent from the information reviewed for this chapter that computers and networked technologies can be used to support and extend professional education in a number of different ways. It has also been emphasized here that confident and competent use of ICT and information management has already become a prerequisite for effective learning and, with the implementation of the NHS Information Strategy, will also be essential for professional practice in the NHS. Although this chapter has focused predominantly on the first steps in the process of promoting effective use of the technology, there is no doubt that clinical educators, and the healthcare professions as a whole, need to take action to incorporate ICT into professional culture. In fact, because higher education institutes have a comparatively long history of using learning technologies, educators could make a valuable contribution by using the resources available to us to promote and support the use of ICT within the healthcare professions.

It has been suggested here that the first steps in promoting the use of these technologies, such as promoting the Web as an information resource, can be made with relatively few adaptations to our teaching (Bonk et al., 1999), but can have very positive outcomes. The evidence from various sources also indicates that specific action to promote and support the development of competence in ICT is the foundation for all future development (Duggleby, 2000; McAvinia and Oliver, 2002; McVay Lynch, 2002). In a similar vein, we have seen that action to incorporate ICT into the existing curriculum can be successfully achieved in stages (Bonk et al., 1999), and that there is growing emphasis on blending computer technologies with traditional face-to-face teaching methods to support flexible learning (Harden and Hart, 2002). In our planning for students, it is feasible to consider that course websites, study packages and/or virtual learning environments could increase the opportunities for flexible learning, especially if this means that more time is made available for face-to-face learning and group discussions when students are on campus.

In many ways, the current uses of multimedia in clinical education are examples of blended learning, because the technology is used as a stimulus for further development of knowledge and skills, through both independent study and class-based discussions. Although relatively few of these multimedia resources are available at present, the evaluations of these (Freeman et al., 1996; Oates and Russell, 1998; Lum and Cox in Chapter 8 of this book) and similar resources by medical educators (Issenberg et al., 2001; Kneebone and ApSimon, 2001) indicate that they can be a valuable complement to traditional approaches to professional and experiential learning. It is feasible to assume that the use of this type of multimedia resource could have a wider role in professional education, especially as changes in the patterns of healthcare delivery are limiting the opportunities for work with some client groups (Friedman, 2000; Kneebone and ApSimon, 2001). This is certainly an area that requires further investigation and possible development in the healthcare professions, as a whole.

This chapter has developed from the recognition that 'the new technologies represent a major societal change, to which clinical educators must respond' (Pickering and McAllister, 1997: 275). As we have seen, there is little doubt that these technologies will play an increasingly important role in professional education and post-qualification activity in the immediate and foreseeable future. Although we are only just beginning to explore how to use these resources, it is clear that our professions and our clients can benefit from further action to harness the technology appropriately.

References

Allan B (2002) E-Learning in the workplace. Information Management Report: The International Newsletter for Information Professionals (May): 1–4.

Anonymous (2001) A funny thing happened on the way to the Web. Law Library Journal 93: 525–528.

Anthony D (2001) Executive Summary of On-line Courses in the Therapies Survey, LTSN. Final report published via Learning and Teaching Support Network – Health Sciences and Practice website. www.health.ltsn.ac.uk/miniproject/completeproj.htm (last accessed 3 March 2003).

ASHA (2002) American Speech-Language-Hearing Association website, www.asha.org/ (last accessed 3 March 2003).

Bader SA, Braude RM (1998) Patient informatics: creating new partnerships in medical decision making. Academic Medicine 73: 408–411.

Ball MJ, Lillis J (2001) E-health: transforming the physician/patient relationship. International Journal of Medical Informatics 61: 1–10.

Bearman M, Cesnick B, Liddell M (2001) Random comparison of 'virtual patient' models in the context of teaching clinical communication skills. Medical Education 35: 824–832.

Bonk CJ, Cummings JA et al. (1999) A ten level Web integration continuum for higher education: new resources, partners, courses, and markets. Available at php.indiana.edu~cjbonk/paper/edmdia99.html (last accessed 3 March 2002). The revised version of this paper appears in Abbey B (ed.) Instructional and Cognitive Impacts of Web-based Education. Hershey, PA: Idea Group Publishing.

Boucher B, Henry J, Hunter D (1999) The effectiveness of computer-assisted instruction in teaching biomechanics of the temporomandibular joint. Journal of Physical Therapy Education 13: 47–81.

Bowen C (2002) members.tripod.com/Caroline_Bowen/home.html (last accessed 3 March 2003).

Brandt KA, Sapp JR, Campbell JM (1996) Current topics in health sciences librarianship: a pilot program for network-based lifelong learning. Bulletin of the Medical Library Association 84: 515–523.

Bryce DA, King NJC, Graebner CF, Myers JH (1998) Exploring student perceptions and addressing faculty concerns. Journal of Interactive Media Education, www-jime.open.ac.uk/98/1/bryce-t.html (last accessed 3 March 2003).

Candy P (2000) Knowledge navigators and lifelong learners: producing graduates for the information society. Higher Education Research and Development 19: 261–277.

Christie A, Wortely P, Jones M (2000) The Internet and clinical reasoning. In Higgs J, Jones ML (eds) Clinical Reasoning in the Health Professions. Oxford: Butterworth Heinemann.

Coles C, Holm HA (1993) Learning in medicine: towards a theory of medical education. In Coles C, Holm HA (eds) Learning in Medicine. Oslo: Scandinavia University Press.

Collins A, Brown JS, Newman S (1989) Cognitive apprenticeship: teaching the crafts of reading, writing and mathematics. In Resnick LB (ed.) Knowing, Learning and Instruction: Essays in Honor of Robert Glaser. Hillsdale, NJ: Lawrence Erlbaum Associates.

Conole G, Oliver M (1998) A pedagogical framework for embedding C&IT into the curriculum. ALT-J (Journal of the Association for Learning and Teaching) 6: 4–16.

Cooper C (2002). Carol Cooper's website: home of the free e-book: the Internet for busy nurses and therapists, www.carol-cooper.co.uk/ (last accessed 3 March 2003).

COT/CSP (1999) The Garner Project: Scoping the Information Management Needs in Occupational Therapy and Physiotherapy. London: College of Occupational Therapists and Chartered Society of Physiotherapists.

COT/CSP (2000) garner@action. London: The College of Occupational Therapists and Chartered Society of Physiotherapists.

Davies ML, Crowther DEA (1995) The benefits of using multimedia in higher education: myths and realities. Active Learning 3: 3–6.

Dearing R (1997). Higher Education in the Learning Society: Report of the National Committee of Enquiry into Higher Education. London: NICHE Publications (HMSO).

DoH (2001) Building the Information Core: Implementing the NHS Plan. London: Department of Health.

DoH (2002). NHS University, www.doh.gov.uk/nhsuniversity/ (last accessed 5 March 2003).

Draper SW, Brown MI, Edgerton E, Henderson FP, McAteer E, Smith ED, Watt HD (1994) Observing and measuring the performance of educational technology. TILT Project Report, c/o Gordon Doughty, Robert Clark Centre, University of Glasgow. Available from the Teaching with Independent Learning Technologies website, www.elec.gla.ac.uk/TILT/TILT/html (last accessed 5 March 2003).

Drew S (1998) Students' perceptions of their learning outcomes. Teaching in Higher Education 3: 197–217.

Duggleby J (2000) How to Be an Online Tutor. London: Gower Publishing.

DxR (2001) Educational Solutions through Technology. Carbondale, IL: DxR Development Group, www.dxrgroup.com/ (last accessed 5 March 2003).

DxR Nursing (2002) Web-based Critical Thinking Software for Nursing Education. Carbondale, IL: DxR Development Group, www.dxrnursing.com/ (last accessed 5 March 2003).

Ericsson KA, Krampe RT, Tesch-Romer C (1993) The role of deliberate practice in the acquisition of expert performance. Psychological Review 100: 363–406.

Ferguson T (2002a) Editorial. From patients to end users. British Medical Journal 324: 555–556.

Ferguson T (2002b) Guidelines for patients. bmj.com (2002).

Freeman M (2001) ViSuAL Voice Version2. Sheffield: Learning Media Unit, University of Sheffield.

Freeman M, Syder D et al. (1996) Bridging the gap between theory and practice: a multimedia tutorial for students of voice therapy. Journal of Voice: Official Journal of the Voice Foundation 10: 292–298.

Friedman CP (2000) The marvellous medical education machine or how medical education can be 'unstuck' in time. Medical Teacher 22: 496–502.

Gagliardi A, Jadad AR (2002) Examination of instruments used to rate quality of health information on the internet: chronicle of a voyage with an unclear destination. British Medical Journal 321: 569–573.

Grabinger RS, Dunlap JC (2000) Rich environments for active learning: a definition. In Squires D, Conole G, Jacobs G (eds) The Changing Face of Learning Technology. Cardiff: University of Wales Press.

Greenhalgh T (2001) Computer assisted learning in undergraduate medical education. British Medical Journal 322: 40–44.

Grimson J, Grimson W, Flahive M, Foley C, O'Moore R, Nolan J, Chadwick G (2000) A multimedia approach to raising awareness of information and communications technology amongst health care professionals. International Journal of Medical Informatics 58/59: 297–305.

Harden RM, Hart IR (2002) An international virtual medical school (IVIMEDS): the future for medical education? Medical Teacher 24: 261–267.

Hasman A (1998) Education and health informatics. International Journal of Medical Informatics 52: 209–216.

Henderson JV (1998) Comprehensive, technology-based clinical education: the 'virtual practicum'. International Journal of Psychiatry in Medicine 28: 41–79.

Hooper C (2002). Welcome to the index page of Web therapy teaching, www.unc.edu/~chooper/classes/voice/webtherapy/index.html (last accessed 3 March 2003).

Horton W (2001) Leading e-learning. Alexandria, VA: ASTD.

Howard S, Perkins M, Martland P (2001) An integrated multi-media package for learning clinical phonetics and linguistics. International Journal of Language & Communication Disorders 36 (supplement): 327–332.

Hughes I, Dewhurst D (2002) Using computer-assisted learning (CAL) software to best effect. Centre for Health Sciences and Practice Newsletter (Learning and Teaching Support Network) (spring): 5–6.

Hulsman RL, Ros WFG, Winnubst JAM, Bensing JM (1999) Teaching clinically experienced physicians communication skills. A review of evaluation studies. Medical Education 33: 655–668.

Hulsman RL, Ros WFG, Winnubst JAM, Bensing JM (2002) The effectiveness of a computer-assisted instruction programme on communication skills of medical specialists in oncology. Medical Education 36: 125–134.

Issenberg SB, Gordon MS, Gordon DL, Safford RE, Hart LR (2001) Simulation and new learning technologies. Medical Teacher 23: 16–23.

JISC (2002) Welcome to the JISC Plagiarism Advisory Service. Information Management Research Institute at Northumbria University. Available at online.northumbria.ac.uk/faculties/art/information_studies/lmri/jiscpas/site/jiscpas.asp (last accessed 5 March 2003).

Kneebone R, ApSimon D (2001) Surgical skills training: simulation and multimedia combined. Medical Education 35: 909–915.

Kolb DA (1984) Experiential Learning: Experience as the Source of Learning and Development. Englewood Cliffs, NJ: Prentice Hall.

Koller C (2000) Twelve tips for developing educational multimedia in a community-based teaching hospital. Medical Teacher 22: 7–10.

Koschman T (1995) Medical education and computer literacy: learning about, through and with computers. Academic Medicine 70: 818–821.

Kunst H, Groot D et al. (2002) Accuracy of information on apparently credible websites: survey of five common health topics. British Medical Journal 321: 581–582.

Kuster J (2002) Net connections for communication disorders and sciences, www.mankato.msus.edu/dept/comdis/kuster2/welcome.html (last accessed 3 March 2003).

Laurillard D (1993) Rethinking University Teaching. London: Routledge.

Laurillard D, McAndrew P (2002) Virtual teaching tools: bringing academics closer to the design of e-learning. Networked Learning 2002: a research based conference on e-learning in higher education and lifelong learning, Sheffield.

Leydon GM, Boulton M, Moynihan C, Jones A, Mossmadn J, Boudioni M, McPherson K (2000) Cancer patients' information needs and information seeking behaviour: an in-depth interview study. British Medical Journal/Information in Practice 320: 909–913.

Liaw T, Kennedy G et al. (2000) Using multimedia to assist students with communication skills and biopsychosocial integration: an evaluation. Australian Journal of Educational Technology 16: 104–125.

Lum C, Cox R (1998) PATSy: a distributed multimedia approach to client assessment skills training. International Journal of Language & Communication Disorders/Royal College of Speech & Language Therapists 33 (supplement): 170–175.

McAteer E, Harris R (2002) Computer-mediated conferencing, LTSN/ALT Resource Guide, leaflet no. 3. Reference no. ELN003. Available from www.ltsn.ac.uk/genericcentre/index.asp?id=17104 (last accessed 3 March 2003).

McAvinia C, Oliver M (2002) 'But my subject's different': a web-based approach to supporting disciplinary lifelong learning skills. Computers and Education 38: 209–220.

McConnell D (2000) Implementing Computer Supported Cooperative Learning. London: Kogan Page.

McVay Lynch M (2002) The Online Educator: A Guide to Creating the Virtual Classroom. London: Routledge Falmer.

Malcomess K (2001) The planning of care. RCSLT Bulletin. 595: 12–13.

MENCAP (2002) MENCAP: understanding learning disability, www.mencap.org.uk (last accessed 3 March 2003).

Milburn A (2001) Foreword. In Building the Information Core – Implementing the NHS Plan. London: Department of Health.

Miller JJ, Piper L, Tucker DA (1997) Strategies for getting students on the information superhighway. Nurse Educator 22(5): 40–43.

NELH (2002) National Electronic Library for Health, NHS, www.nelh.nhs.uk/ (last accessed 3 March 2003).

NINDS (2002) National Institute for Neurological Disorders and Stroke, www.ninds.nih.gov/ (last accessed 3 March 2003).

NMAP (2002) The Internet for Allied Health, nmap.ac.uk (last accessed 3 March 2003).

Oates J, Russell A (1998) Learning voice analysis using an interactive multi-media package: development and preliminary evaluation. Journal of Voice: Official Journal of the Voice Foundation 12: 500–512.

OFSTED (2002) ICT in Schools: Effect of Government Initiatives. London: Office for Standards in Education.

O'Leary R (2002) Virtual learning environments, LTSN Generic Centre/ALT.

PATSy (2003) Welcome to the PATSy website: database for teaching and research. Available at www.patsy.ac.uk/main.html (last accessed 3 March 2003).

Phipps R, Merisotis J (1999) What's the difference? A review of contemporary research on the effectiveness of distance learning in higher education. Institute for Higher Education Policy at the behest of the American Federation of Teachers and National Education Association.

Pickering M, McAllister S (1997) Clinical education and the future: an emerging mosaic of change, challenge and creativity. In McAllister L, Lincoln M, McLeod S, Maloney D (eds) Facilitating Learning in Clinical Settings. Cheltenham: Stanley Thornes.

Purcell GP, Wilson P et al. (2002) Editorial. The quality of health information on the internet. British Medical Journal 324: 557–558.

RCSLT (2002) Royal College of Speech and Language Therapists website, www.rcslt.org (last accessed 3 March 2003).

Reingold H (1995) The Virtual Community. London: Minerva.

RNID (2002) RNID for deaf and hard of hearing people website, www.rnid.org.uk (last accessed 3 March 2003).

Roberts JM, Copeland KL (2001) Clinical websites are dangerous to health. International Journal of Medical Informatics 62: 181–187.

Russell AL (1995) Stages in learning new technology: naive adult email users. Computers & Education 25: 173–178.

Salmon S (2000) E-Moderating: The Key to Teaching and Learning Online. London: Kogan Page.

Schön DA (1987) Educating the Reflective Practitioner: Toward a New Design for Teaching and Learning in the Professions. San Francisco, CA: Jossey-Bass.

Staggers N, Gassert CA, Skiba DJ (2000) Health professionals' views of informatics education: findings from the AMIA 1999 Spring Conference. Journal of the American Medical Informatics Association 7: 550–558.

Steele DJ, Palensky JEJ, Lynch TG, Lacy NL, Duffy SW (2002) Learning preferences, computer attitudes, and student evaluation of computerised instruction. Medical Education 36: 225–232.

Stubley P (2002) What's yours is mine. Information Management Report: The International Newsletter for Information Professionals (August): 1–4.

Tait B (1997) Constructive Internet based learning. Active Learning 7 (December): 3–7.

Timms D, Crompton P, Booth S, Allen P (1997) The implementation of learning technologies: the experience of Project Varsetile. Active Learning 6 (July): 3–9.

Treadwell I, de Witt TW, Grobler S (2002) The impact of a new educational strategy on acquiring neonatology skills. Medical Education 36: 441–448.

Vogel M, Wood DF (2002) Love it or hate it? Medical attitudes to computer-assisted learning. Medical Education 36: 214–215.

Wang F-K, Bonk CJ (2001) A design framework for electronic cognitive apprenticeship. Journal of Asynchronous Learning Networks 5: 131–151.

Watson B (2001) Key factors affecting conceptual gains from CAL materials. British Journal of Educational Technology 32: 587–593.

Wilson H (2001) The Old Geezer's Toolbox for Speech Therapy, www.tcsn.net/geezer/HOME.HTM#index2 (last accessed 3 March 2003).

Wilson P (2002) How to find the good and avoid the bad or ugly: a short guide to tools for rating quality of health information on the internet. British Medical Journal 324: 598–600.

Ziv A, Samall SD, Wolpe PR (2000) Patient safety and simulation-based medical education. Medical Teacher 22: 489–495.

Chapter 8
Case-based teaching and clinical reasoning: seeing how students think with PATSy

Richard Cox and Carmel Lum

Introduction

This chapter introduces PATSy (www.patsy.ac.uk) – a web-based multimedia database shell that has been designed to accept data from any discipline that has cases. PATSy makes 'virtual patients' available to trainees, educators and researchers in various clinical professions and cognate academic disciplines. The systems contain 61 data-rich and extensively described cases of adults and children with disorders that can be accessed under four domain headings: speech and language, dyslexia, medical rehabilitation and neuropsychology. PATSy functions as both an archive for research and clinical cases and a community resource.

The chapter includes a brief history on the development of PATSy, together with a description of a typical student user session. The roles that PATSy can play in speech and language therapy education are also discussed. Different methods of teaching with PATSy and examples of how PATSy supports didactic, case-based and problem-based methods of teaching and learning in speech and language therapy are provided. The use of PATSy as a research tool for studying clinical reasoning and problem solving is described and illustrated with examples from an investigation of student reasoning. It is argued that PATSy can act as a bridge between research and education and between research and clinical practice.

Trends in professional education

Professional education is turning increasingly towards case-based teaching where knowledge of the subject is represented in the form of many example cases that embody the relevant principles (e.g. Irby, 1994). This method and variants of it are advocated in the teaching of knowledge-intensive domains such as medicine and law. In those domains it is difficult to give the student a set of rules that they may use to make inferences or deductions (Williams, 1993; Jonassen, 1996). In case-based reasoning, students acquire a mental library of cases from which to reason (Riesbeck and Schank, 1991; Kolodner, 1993). A case that has features analogous to those of the current problem is retrieved and used as a basis for reasoning about the new situation – in other words, old solutions are adapted and applied to new problems. A related approach is termed 'problem-based learning', in which several individual students study the same case and then engage in educational activities such as group discussions with a facilitator (Barrows, 1985; Jonassen, 1996). Hmelo (1995) has shown that medical students taught using problem-based learning produce more accurate diagnostic hypotheses than non-problem-based learning students.

In recent years, there has been a theoretical shift in some speech and language courses – from a 'medical model' in which the purpose of assessment was to derive taxonomic classification, to a new approach based on information-processing (IP) accounts of language processing (Ellis and Young, 1996; Stackhouse and Wells, 1997). IP accounts of language are based on normal experimental and cognitive neuropsychological evidence in which language disorders are seen in terms of an impairment to normal representations and processes. Language assessment is based on a cognitive neuropsychological model and is motivated by hypotheses developed through a knowledge of psycholinguistic theories of language and cognition.

Cognitive neuropsychological analysis of language disorders is one example of a theory-driven or rule-based approach in which models of normal language, abnormal language and cognition are used to guide assessment, diagnosis and treatment.

The traditional approach (i.e. categorization of patients according to syndromes) can be thought of as one that entails inductive reasoning – looking for patterns among the test scores by which to classify patients. In contrast, the IP-based approach requires hypothesis-driven, deductive reasoning.

In learning to diagnose deductively, students are encouraged to learn rules (theory) and apply these in their selection of suitable tests for the patient and how to utilize the results of a pre-existing test to inform the selection of subsequent tests – all in the pursuit of verifying an initial hypothesis. Novices, despite the absence of clinical experience and mastery of the domain, can achieve success in a rule-based approach.

Later, when the student has attained greater levels of competence and experience, he or she may find himself or herself better able to reason and make sense of large amounts of data. Inductive reasoning is more intuitive for most people than deduction and it tends to predominate in everyday thinking (Robertson, 1999). However, in a clinical context, a novice presented with an amassed collection of information about a patient lacks the background knowledge and clinical experience required to reason validly in an inductive mode. Consequently PATSy offers a means by which to develop rule-based, deductive approaches to test selection by allowing the controlled and systematic revelation of information as testing proceeds. This potential of computer-based systems in case-based teaching is becoming increasingly recognized (Schank, 1991; Edelson, 1996; Jonassen, 1996).

PATSy in professional education: what challenges does PATSy address?

- **Changes in educational teaching methods:** education in the health professions is turning increasingly towards case-based teaching where subject knowledge is represented in the form of many example cases.
- **Provision of access to people with speech and language disorders for clinical training:** clinical science students traditionally receive clinical skills training during placements in hospitals and community centres. This, of course, is an important and vital part of their training. However, there are often problems with access to suitable training experiences. Even where people with disorders are available, the quality of a student's experience in acquiring clinical assessment knowledge depends on the type and variety of patients available during their placement period. For these reasons, some students' assessment experiences, knowledge of various speech disorders, etc., may be acquired on a somewhat ad hoc basis. It is, of course, desirable for students to have access to patient cases prior to clinical placement – this is where PATSy is invaluable.
- **Pre-clinical training and rehearsal opportunities:** under current regimes of clinical training, students usually do not have any interactions with people with communication disorders until they are on clinical placement. It would, of course, be more desirable for students to have access to patient cases prior to this time. They would then: (a) be familiar with an adequate range of speech disorders, and (b) have more technical knowledge of assessment before meeting 'live' patients. Students also need to practise and hone their diagnostic skills, but ethical considerations often prevent them from practising assessments repeatedly on the same patient. Furthermore, even in clinics, patients may not always be available, as medical care takes priority over training. A further point is that students have little control over when and where they can practise assessment procedures because traditional training is bound to the clinic schedule.
- **Providing opportunity for private and extended practice ('learning by doing'):** students need to learn about assessment tests and to practise diagnosis. However, ethical considerations often deprive them of opportunities for practising assessments repeatedly on the same patient. PATSy allows them to practise as much as they want – virtual patients do not complain or tire!

- **Access to rare cases:** PATSy contains some rare cases.
- **Interprofessionality:** PATSy attempts to bridge the chasms between disciplines by providing access to cases in other disciplines (for example medicine, psychology and special education).
- **Assessment:** with traditional clinic-based training placements, educators cannot assume that their students have seen similar patient cases. With PATSy, though, a whole class can experience and discuss the same cases and can be set a 'virtual' patient to diagnose under exam conditions.
- **Internet access:** PATSy is accessible via the Internet (Web) and hence is available to a wide range of users whenever needed.
- **Support for various approaches to teaching** including case-based teaching, problem-based learning, student-based guided exploratory learning and traditional lectures.
- **Provision of a standardized corpus of cases** against which each student's performance may be appraised, allows students to engage in assessment training independently of the clinic setting and at times convenient to the student.
- **Researchers' facility for publishing material** supplementary to that included in journal articles; space limitations can be overcome when researchers place extensive data on PATSy (19 out of 21 cases in PATSy speech and language therapy have featured in published research papers).

An introduction to PATSy and a brief history of its development

PATSy (www.patsy.ac.uk; Lum and Cox, 1998; Lum et al., 1999) is an Internet-based multimedia database system that provides 'virtual' patient cases for students in the clinical sciences such as clinical psychology, speech and language therapy, medicine and related fields. This chapter focuses on PATSy's speech and language domain content, but the system is a generic database shell that has been designed to accept multimedia and data from any discipline that has cases.

PATSy originated as the result of a collaboration between the two authors in the mid-1990s. The aim was to re-purpose or re-use a collection of research-grade (i.e. extensively tested patients) case data which existed in the form of video and audio tapes, and paper-based records. This PATSy 'seed' data had been collected in the course of research on non-propositional ('automatic') aphasic speech by the second author at the University of York (Lum and Ellis, 1999). The initial plan was to produce interactive CD-ROMs and a prototype was developed. However, following the rapid development of the World Wide Web and viable

PC-based hypermedia browsers, it quickly became clear that the Web offered a feasible and better alternative. A Web-based approach offers many advantages over CD-ROM for a system such as PATSy, such as the ability to centrally update the system for all users simultaneously, platform independence for users (i.e. usable on PCs, Macintoshes, etc.), ability to control and manage access, variety of multimedia formats, etc. Although video and other large multimedia files make high demands on computer networks, it was realized that the (immediate) potential users of PATSy were based in UK tertiary institutions, and would therefore have Janet/SuperJanet (fast broadband) access to the Internet. (The clinical sector is also beginning to enjoy broadband Internet access with the recent advent of NHSNet; www.nhsia.nhs.uk)

A successful proposal to the Nuffield Foundation (a UK charitable foundation) allowed the first PATSy project to begin 1998 as a collaboration between the universities of Edinburgh, York, Newcastle-upon-Tyne and Queen Margaret University College. The first development project produced a multimedia collection of test and case data from adults and children with speech and language disorders. A second round of funding by the Nuffield Foundation followed, and the second PATSy project saw a collaboration between the universities of Sussex, York and Cambridge, and the Astley Ainslie Rehabilitation Hospital (Edinburgh) which resulted in three further domains being added to the system – dyslexia, neuropsychology and medical rehabilitation (in April 2002). Currently, the system contains 61 cases and 556 tests, many including digital video and audio recordings, International Phonetic Alphabet (IPA) transcriptions of patient responses and other rich multimedia representations. Twenty-one of the cases are categorized as speech and language (Table 8.1). A further domain (audiology) is in the process of being developed.

PATSY is designed to be a raw data archive of case data from either research or demonstration cases and may include clinical and non-clinical participants. It is useful as a resource for storing 'rare' case data, as well as a means of illustrating typical cases. Specifically, PATSy is intended to be an archive that interfaces research with education and practice. The system was developed to provide a useful resource for clinicians and researchers and an interactive learning environment in which students can develop their clinical reasoning skills.

The system is presently in use by over 20 UK university departments (speech and language therapy, psychology, medicine). Eighty percent of UK speech and language therapy departments use the system. It offers educators and researchers a facility for disseminating material to students and supports the dissemination of research by offering researchers a facility for storing interactive multimedia representations of their data (i.e. serving as a rich appendix to published journal papers).

Table 8.1 PATSy speech and language cases.

Patient	Description	Disability	Case type
AER	Sentence-processing intervention	Syntax	Research
AL	Syntactic problems	Syntax	Research
AZ	Child language	Semantic, syntax	Demonstration
BK	Lexical access problems in speech production	Lexical	Research
BS	Surface dyslexia	Reading	Research
CB	Word-sound deafness with syntactic problems	Auditory	Demonstration
CC	Right-hemisphere discourse problems	Discourse	Demonstration
DB	Lexical access and syntactic problems in speech production	Lexical, syntax	Research
DBL	Lexical access problems in speech production with recurrent speech	Lexical	Research
DrO	Word-meaning deafness	Auditory	Research
EA	Parkinson's – prosodic comprehension problems	Auditory	Research
IB	Speech-processing and reading problems (deep dyslexia)	Lexical, auditory, syntax, reading	Research
JG	Sentence processing, reading and anomia	Syntax, reading	Research
JS	Word-sound deafness with other language problems	Auditory	Research
JW	Auditory memory problem	Auditory	Research
LY	Dysarthria – Wilson's disease	Motor speech	Demonstration
MSL	Severe form of lexical problems in speech production	Lexical	Research
NH	Lexical access problems in speech production and auditory processing deficits	Lexical, auditory	Research
NM	Lexical access problems in speech production with foreign accent syndrome	Lexical	Demonstration
RN	Child phonology	Auditory	Demonstration
TB	Parkinson's – prosodic comprehension problems	Auditory	Research

Reports and focus group evaluations (see www.patsy.ac.uk/speech/reports.html) indicate that students and tutors find the system useful. Feedback comments include:

- 'Helps in placement with patients – particularly in clinics where it gives the student more confidence.'
- 'Could help in planning patient assessment.'
- 'Helps in developing hypotheses.'
- 'Helps you feel more confident – doing a test in PATSy rather than with a real patient. Can repeat the test.'
- 'Having the references is extremely useful.'
- 'It allows you to test your hypotheses quickly, rather than waiting for the next appointment with a patient!'

- 'It familiarizes students with tests, and clinicians with tests they may not see within their clinic, e.g. new tests, research tests, etc. This may be especially useful for students if they are in a placement where they are not seeing many tests.'

PATSy is indexed in numerous reviewed Internet directories and portals (see www.patsy.ac.uk/plinks.html) including the UK government's 'National Grid for Learning'.

Educators may 'personalize' PATSy content by submitting their own references, demonstration cases, tutorial questions and comments about any of the cases on the system. These kinds of contribution can be shared with other users nationally or reserved for local use. Researchers may also submit case data and multimedia material to support their reports of cases in journal publications (as a kind of online appendix). PATSy also provides a research tool for investigating student diagnostic reasoning – this use of PATSy will be discussed further below.

PATSy patient case categorization

Of the 21 speech and language therapy cases on PATSy, 15 are 'research' cases and six are 'demonstration' cases (Table 8.1). It is recognized that the requirements for rigour and detail in research and education respectively do vary in some contexts and the categorization of PATSy cases into demonstration and research cases is intended to capture these differences.

Demonstration case-type

This category is intended to refer to contributions that demonstrate one or any of a behavioural event, a clinical procedure or an assessment. The material may be too sparse to serve research but offers educators examples for illustrative or demonstration purposes.

Some uses of a demonstration case might be to illustrate:

- how to administer and interpret a particular test
- the difference between flaccid and spastic dysarthria
- how to conduct a clinical interview with a depressed patient.

Research case-type

The participant's material may be categorized as a research case according to some or all of these criteria:

- The participant's disorder has been comprehensively described by normed tests or tasks such that other researchers may reanalyse the data (i.e. useful for data extraction by users accessing PATSy in data mode).
- The quality of the data is good, i.e. the data are clear and intelligible. Rigorous methods of data collection are employed.

- The participant is reported in a published journal paper as a single case study, case series or a group study.

Research cases serve to archive data, which is especially useful to the speech and language therapy community if the participant represents a rare or unusual case but is useful too for 'typical' cases. This kind of case can also supplement a journal publication by storing the participant's raw data on PATSy as an extended appendix for journal readers to consult. Research cases can, of course, be used as demonstration cases, but not vice versa.

Sustainability, ethics and security

The ethos of PATSy is that of a shared resource which is used, maintained and contributed to by members of the speech and language therapy community. The project aims to provide a high-quality, secure (password-protected, etc.) facility for communicating and sharing information among and between educators and researchers.

In the UK, PATSy's longer-term sustainability is based on a non-profit subscription model. Users pay an annual subscription fee (note that a PATSY 'user' is an academic or teaching hospital department, not an individual). Subscription revenue pays for programming, support, hardware/software updates and for subsidizing workshop attendance. Workshops are held periodically to introduce PATSy to new users or provide user training for specific functions such as data installation.

Neurological test results, medical and case histories are available for all cases on the system. The medical histories are actual medical histories except that the names of the patient, medical personnel and relatives, and any private information are concealed or altered.

Informed patient consent for the use of data in PATSy has been obtained. Authorization for use of copyright test material has also been obtained. Numerous precautions have been undertaken to protect patients' privacy and to comply with the terms of the consent provided by the patient. The PATSy website is secure and accessible only by username and password and by users accessing the system from academic Internet domains. Access codes are allocated to users by designated local administrators in each subscribing department. All users are required to read and agree to be bound by PATSy's conditions of use when they first access the system.

What PATSy is not

It might be useful to point out how PATSy differs from other kinds of computer-based educational resource. PATSy is not designed as an information resource for consultation by the public, nor is PATSy a computer-based tutor that teaches via direct instruction according to some internally represented curriculum. No particular educational approach is embodied in the system. It is designed to be a flexible resource for use in a variety of educational and research situations.

Interacting with the system – a sample student session

The system contains data from numerous speech and language-disordered patients (Table 8.1). Each case is represented using multimedia, which typically includes digitized video clip(s) of the patient speaking with the therapist, recordings of the patient undergoing a range of assessment tests, and interactive multimedia clips showing test items and patient responses to test stimuli.

A typical student interaction with PATSy might proceed as follows: using a web browser such as Microsoft's Internet Explorer or Netscape Navigator, the student logs onto PATSy with a personal password (Figure 8.1).

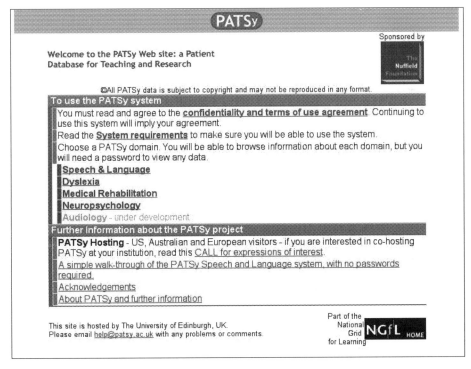

Figure 8.1 The PATSy welcome page.

The student then selects the 'Speech & Language' domain (Figure 8.1). Clicking on 'Student', the student goes to the PATSy speech and language home page (Figure 8.2) and selects the kind of cases needed (Figure 8.3) on the basis of 'Age Group' – options 'adult', 'child', 'either'; 'Time' – 'single assessment', 'longitudinal', 'therapy'; and 'Case Type' – 'research', 'demonstration', 'either', using drop-down menus. The student can also set 'Logging' to 'on' or 'off'. 'Assessment Practice' and 'Information Only' modes are described in the 'Other modes of accessing PATSy' section below.

PATSy

PATSy Speech & Language Home Page

Welcome to the home page for the PATSy Speech and Language web site.

Select a mode of entry to PATSy from the list below. You will require an appropriate username and password for each mode. For password information, please contact your local PATSy administrator.

Alternatively you can browse the information on this PATSy domain by clicking on the links in the lower panel.

Please contact help@patsy.ac.uk to report any problems or simply to comment on the system.

PATSy Modes
- Guest
- Student
- Examination
- Researcher / Clinician
- Data Mode
- Administrator

More Information on PATSy Speech & Language
- Acknowledgements
- Cases on PATSy Speech & Language
- Walkthrough - a simple walkthrough of PATSy Speech & Language with no passwords required
- PATSy Speech & Language - Specialist Team Details
- Feedback Reports
- Induction to PATSy Speech & Language - we suggest this as a useful introduction for students using PATSy.

Home

Figure 8.2 PATSy Speech & Language domain home page.

PATSy

PATSy User Options

Select options below, then press the *Go To Patients* button, to go to a list of patients.

User Options

Change the patient properties to determine which patients are selected from the PATSy database. The logging option determines whether you will be requested to add to the log by posting your thoughts periodically. The *type* option allows you to select different modes of access to PATSy: *assessment practise* presents cases for you to test your assessment skills, whereas *information only* provides more background and scoring information on the cases.

Patient Properties				Session Properties	
Age Group	**Time**	**Case Type**		**Logging**	**Type**
○ Child				● No Logging	● Assessment Practise
○ Adult	any	Research		○ Logging	○ Information Only
● Either	Single				
	Longitudinal				
	Therapy				
	any				

Go To Patients

Home

Figure 8.3 Selecting required case type in Student mode.

The student would then typically go on to select a patient from a menu of cases returned by the search (Figure 8.4).

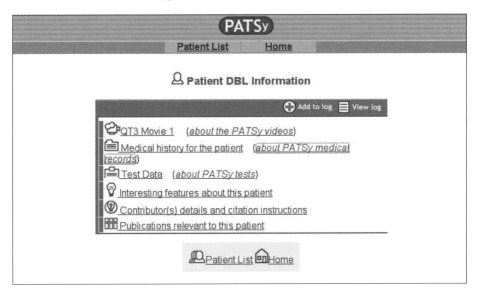

> ⚐ **Patient List**
>
> This is the list of patients fitting your criteria who are currently present in the PATSy database. All patients will primarily be known by these two or three letter identifiers. Patients' real names are never disclosed.
>
> ⚐ AER
> ⚐ AL
> ⚐ AZ
> ⚐ BK
> ⚐ BS
> ⚐ CB
> ⚐ CC
> ⚐ DB
> ⚐ DBL
> ⚐ DrO
> ⚐ EA
> ⚐ IB
> ⚐ JG

Figure 8.4 List of cases selected.

Selecting case 'DBL', the user is presented with a list of options (Figure 8.5). At this point students typically observe video clips of the patient speaking or read the medical history. The student may then be required to formulate a clinical hypothesis based on initial observations.

> **PATSy**
>
> Patient List   Home
>
> ⚐ **Patient DBL Information**
>
> ➕ Add to log ☰ View log
>
> 📹 QT3 Movie 1   (*about the PATSy videos*)
> 📖 Medical history for the patient   (*about PATSy medical records*)
> 🗒 Test Data   (*about PATSy tests*)
> 💡 Interesting features about this patient
> Ⓥ Contributor(s) details and citation instructions
> ▦ Publications relevant to this patient
>
> ⚐ Patient List 🏠 Home

Figure 8.5 Options for case 'DBL'.

Next, the student would typically go to the test list for the patient (DBL in this case). Tests can then be 'administered' to the patient by selecting the desired test from a structured menu (Figure 8.6).

📧 Tests administered for patient DBL

Educational Support
IPA Charts
Types of test scores explained

➕ Add to log   📋 View log

Test	Max. Total	Correct Score	Proportion correct
ADA L1: Lexical Decision (spoken)	160	143	.89
ADA L1Wr: Lexical Decision (written)	160	142	.89
ADA L2Wr: Reading of Words	80	65	.81
ADA P1: Minimal Pairs same voice nonwords	40	39	.98
ADA P2: Minimal Pairs different voice non-words	40	29	.73
ADA RWr: Nonword Reading	40	20	.50
Howard & Franklin 100 pictures: Naming	100	68	.68
Howard & Franklin 100 pictures: Reading	100	90	.90
Howard & Franklin 100 pictures: Repeating	100	100	1
Nonword and Word Repetition	80	73	.91
Palpa 49: Synonym Judgement (spoken)	60	47	.67
Palpa 50: Synonym Judgement (written)	60	46	.77
Pyramids and Palm Trees (picture-picture condition)	52	47	.90
Pyramids and Palm Trees (picture-word condition)	52	43	.83
Pyramids and Palm Trees (word-word condition)	52	38	.73
Short-term digit recall (auditory)		3.75	
Short-term digit recall (visual)		3	
Short-term matching span (auditory)		4	
Short-term matching span (visual)		3	
TROG (spoken)	20	11 blocks	
Western Aphasia Battery	100	82.7	827

Figure 8.6 Test list for case 'DBL' (NB as seen by Research users – the score summary table is not provided to Student users – they see a list of test names only).

Netscape: Log for patsy about patient NH

Access: Patient NH Information page [Sun Oct 4 17:21:53 BST 1998]

Access: Medical record for patient NH [Sun Oct 4 17:24:25 BST 1998]

Access: Tutorial Questions on Medical Record for patient NH [Sun Oct 4 17:24:44 BST 1998]

User Notes:

- **Conclusions?**: This patient ahd a stroke about 8 years ago. She appears to have no difficulty folloiwng conversation though she has considerable problems trying to speak. her major problem appears to be in speech production.
- **Where next?**: I would like to carry-out an all-over check on her auditory comprehension to eliminate the possibility that she might have comprehension problems (however, minor). My choice of test would be the TROG.
- **Why?**: The TROG is a test of syntax comprehension but it also provides an indication of the patient's abiltiy to comprehend single words (nouns, adjectives, prepositions) as well as cope with varying lengths of sentences.

Access: Patient NH Information page [Sun Oct 4 17:31:42 BST 1998]

Access: Test List [Sun Oct 4 17:31:45 BST 1998]

Access: Test TROG (spoken) - sentences [Sun Oct 4 17:31:50 BST 1998]
Single test item accesses for the above test:
1,2,3,4,5,6,7,8,9,10,11,12,13,14,15,16,17,18,19,20,21,22,23,24,25,
26,27,28,29,30,31,32,33,34,35,36,37,38,39,40,41,42,43,44,45,46,
47,48,49,50,,51,52,53,54,55,56,57,58,59,60,61,62,63,64
Access: Patient NH Information page [Sun Oct 4 17:32:47 BST 1998]

User Notes:

- **Conclusions?**: The patient passed 11 blocks though the norm for elderly patients is 14 blocks. She as a minor comprehension problem though this is not attributable to the comprehension of content words. There is no particular error pattern to suggest its a syntactic problem so it maybe that she has a STM deficit.
- **Where next?**: I'd like to asess NH in auditory STM
- **Why?**: If NH has auditory STM problems this could account for her failing the blocks with longer sentences.

Figure 8.7 Example of student reflective comments interleaved with PATSy-generated log data.

No.	Stimulus (audio)	Stimulus (text)	Class	Response (audio)	Transcript of patient response	Score
					Test date: 27th January 1993	Add to log
1	Listen to Stimulus	/dʒb/	b	Listen to Response	/dʒb/	1
2	Listen to Stimulus	wear	a	Listen to Response	wear	1
3	Listen to Stimulus	patience	c	Listen to Response	patience	1
4	Listen to Stimulus	/bæsfəl/	d	Listen to Response	/bæsfəl/	1
5	Listen to Stimulus	bishop	c	Listen to Response	bishop	1
6	Listen to Stimulus	act	a	Listen to Response	act	1
7	Listen to Stimulus	/mʌnkɒm/	d	Listen to Response	/mʌnkɒm/	1
8	Listen to Stimulus	/keɪ/	b	Listen to Response	/keɪ/	1
9	Listen to Stimulus	doctor	c	Listen to Response	doctor	1
10	Listen to Stimulus	/rɒdɪn/	d	Listen to Response	/rʌdɪn/	0
11	Listen to Stimulus	moth	a	Listen to Response	/mɒθ/	0
12	Listen to Stimulus	/baɪʃ/	b	Listen to Response	/baɪʃ/	1
13	Listen to Stimulus	task	a	Listen to Response	task	1
14	Listen to Stimulus	stomach	c	Listen to Response	stomach	1
15	Listen to Stimulus	/ʃrævəl/	d	Listen to Response	/ʃrævəl/	1
16	Listen to Stimulus	/hæt/	b	Listen to Response	/hæt/	1
17	Listen to Stimulus	cure	a	Listen to Response	cure	1
18	Listen to Stimulus	/dræn/	b	Listen to Response	/dræn/	1
19	Listen to Stimulus	forbid	c	Listen to Response	forbid	1
20	Listen to Stimulus	/stupɪm/	d	Listen to Response	/stjupɪm/	1

Figure 8.8 Example of IPA transcription of patient response to ADA test items.

Throughout a PATSy training session students are encouraged to state their model-derived hypotheses in advance, to reflect on their conclusions and to state explicitly what they plan to do next based on those conclusions (Figure 8.7). If the student set logging to 'on' at the case selection stage (Figure 8.3), then the student will be periodically prompted to type in responses to reflective questions: 'Conclusions so far?', 'Where next?' and 'Why?'. Where appropriate, PATSy displays IPA transcriptions of patient utterances (Figure 8.8).

When accessed in student assessment mode, each case consists of a medical history, video clip(s) and assessment data. A wide range of test data is available for each patient. On average, each case on PATSy Speech & Language contains 27 tests. This represents rich 'research-grade' data for each case on the system. Students can step through any test item by item. For example, in a test where the clinician presents auditory stimuli, the student can listen to a digitized audio clip of a clinician presenting the items to the patient, followed by digitized audio clips of the patient's actual responses to those items. The student records the patient's test results on the test score sheet, as if the student were actually in a clinic. In light of the test data, the student may revise his or her initial clinical hypothesis, with the process continuing until the student is satisfied that sufficient information to diagnose the source of the patient's speech and language problem has been acquired. An example is provided by 'TROG' test item 67 (Figure 8.9). In the case of the representation of the TROG on PATSy, the student can play a sound file of the (spoken) stimulus (in this case the sentence 'Not only the girl, but also the cat, is sitting') and then click on a second button to reveal the picture that the patient pointed to in response to the stimulus (depicted by an animated arrow; Figure 8.9).

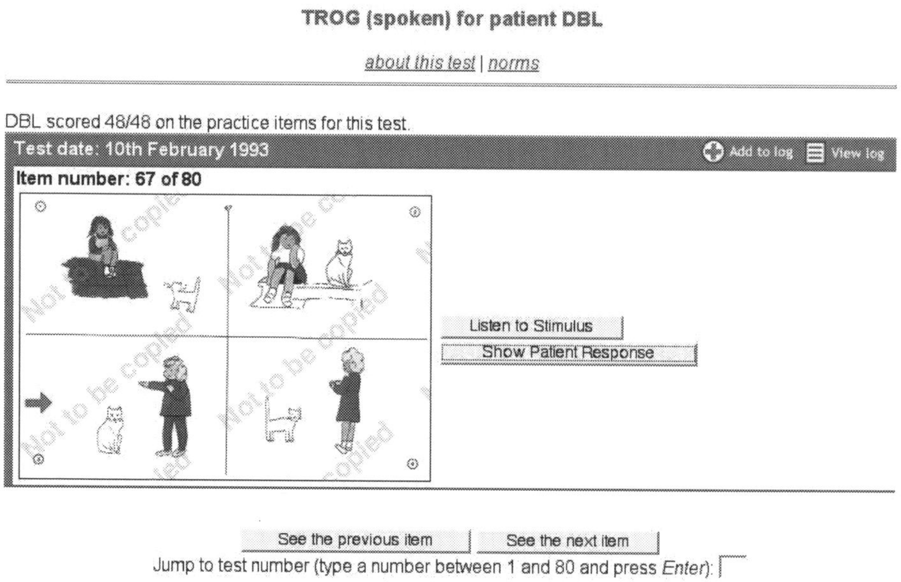

TROG (spoken) for patient DBL

about this test | norms

DBL scored 48/48 on the practice items for this test.

Test date: 10th February 1993   ⊕ Add to log ▤ View log

Item number: 67 of 80

Listen to Stimulus
Show Patient Response

See the previous item   See the next item

Jump to test number (type a number between 1 and 80 and press *Enter*):

Figure 8.9 Item from the test of reception of grammar (TROG; Bishop, 1989). The user can click the 'Listen to stimulus' button and hear the spoken stimulus ('Not only the girl, but also the cat, is sitting'), and can then reveal which picture the patient pointed to by pressing the 'Show patient response' button – an arrow is then revealed alongside one of the stimuli as shown in the lower left picture (NB the patient made an error on this item).

Diary feature

As mentioned above, PATSy records the sequence of clinical testing by the student. A note-taking facility for users is also provided. The notepad feature is invoked by pressing the 'Add to log' button (this button can be seen in Figures 8.5, 8.6, 8.8 and 8.9). Following a PATSy session, the student can save or print out the test log. This can later act as a stimulus for discussions between the tutor and his or her student in a problem-based learning session. Text typed into the prompt fields by the student is interleaved with machine-generated log data and stored for later retrieval. The student's notes are automatically interleaved with machine-generated user-system information as shown in Figure 8.7. Prompting occurs at fixed time intervals or on moving from one test to another. Alternatively, students can record their reflections at any time by clicking on the 'Add to log' button.

Other modes of accessing PATSy

The example above illustrated one use of PATSy by a student in 'student information only' mode. PATSy offers numerous other modes of access:

- guest
- student (sub-modes = 'assessment' and 'information only')
- examination
- researcher/clinician
- data mode
- administrator.

Extensive educational support material is provided on PATSY but it is separated from case content and made available to users via 'educational support' links. Examples of educational support material include tutorial questions for students and reference material on tests prepared by tutors for their students to refer to. Examples of links to educational support material can be seen in Figure 8.6. The induction guide for students (www.patsy.ac.uk/speech/induction.html) is another example.

Student assessment practice mode

This is the mode in which the illustrative student–PATSy interaction described above took place. It is typically used by students in clinical training. It is one of two student modes and provides an opportunity for fine-grained, item-by-item administration of tests to patients. Students can 'administer' tests to the patient then score and interpret patient performance. This mode is particularly useful for practising the administration of unfamiliar tests before meeting 'live' patients.

By design, this mode provides a relatively minimal amount of patient information to the student. The aim is to maintain the student's focus on test administration, interpretation of results and generating hypotheses.

Student information mode

In student information mode, the user can progress through test items on an item-by-item basis (as in student assessment mode). However, the following additional information is also provided:

- the patient data contributor's contact details
- publications relevant to the patient/disorder
- interesting features about the patient's disorder.

A search facility is available to student information and researcher-level users which enables searches for particular tests, types of patient, particular responses or stimuli, etc.

Exam mode

Cases can be held back by tutors for use as unseen patients for purposes of student assessment. Exam mode provides similar information to student information mode, but is intended to involve assessment of a patient the student has not previously seen on PATSy.

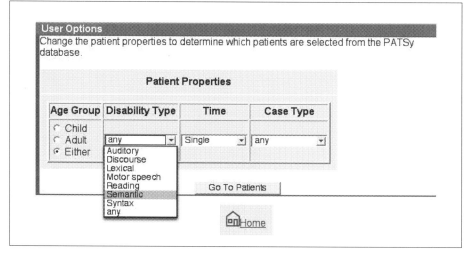

Figure 8.10 Selecting required case type in Researcher mode.

Researcher mode

This is the 'deluxe' level of access to PATSy's database and is typically used by researchers and clinicians rather than students. It presents the user with test summary tables (total scores for all the tests a given patient has undertaken, as shown in Figure 8.6).

The researcher mode is suited to users who come with considerable background knowledge and experience that guides their interpretation of such a mass of data. However, those educators who prefer a traditional (taxonomic) approach to diagnostics would probably be more inclined to offer their students researcher mode than student mode. Researcher mode encompasses all the levels of performance description available in both types of student mode. A search facility allows searches to be made for particular tests, types of patient, particular responses or stimuli, etc.

Users in researcher mode can select cases on a different basis than that provided in student modes, i.e. that of disorder type (compare Figures 8.3 and 8.10).

Other modes

'Guest' mode is a restricted mode of access designed to allow potential PATSy subscribers and other interested parties to explore PATSy in a way that avoids the need for formal conditions-of-use-agreements to be signed. In guest mode, information is presented as for student information mode, but only one patient is available. In addition, a non-patient video clip is substituted for the patient video to comply with PATSy's terms and conditions of use. Another type of access (data mode) provides a facility for exporting raw test data in a form suitable for use in a spreadsheet or as input to a statistical package such as SPSS.

In 'data' mode, when a test list for a PATSy case is accessed (as in Figure 8.6), each test has an 'extract' button to the left of its name. Clicking an extract button causes a data file consisting of rows/columns of test item names, scores, etc., to be downloaded to the user's PC. This facility was developed in response to requests by PATSy users interested in using PATSy data as training set input for computational models, and for use in training students in statistical analysis.

Finally, 'administrator' mode allows local administrators in subscribing departments to perform housekeeping functions, such as issuing student accounts (singly or in groups), selecting which patients local users can access, holding back patients for use in student examinations, specifying their local users' modes of access, setting which tests their local users 'see' for each case, etc. Administrators can also monitor their local users' interaction logs to ensure appropriate use of the system. A facility for PATSy users to contribute new patient and test content of their own is also available from within this mode.

PATSy and research in professional education

PATSy has numerous potential roles in research:

- as a tool for collecting data on student reasoning
- making it easier for patient data to be re-examined by different researchers
- allowing existing data to be reconsidered in light of new theoretical developments
- allowing researchers to relate their research patients to similar patients reported in the literature
- allowing researchers to test new hypotheses on the data presented by PATSy patients.

These are quite general research roles, but PATSy can be used to conduct research on clinical reasoning that would be quite difficult to do in traditional contexts. An example of this is provided by a recent study of clinical reasoning (Cox and Lum, 2003), described below. PATSy's research features include a student–system interaction recording and student diary facility and the 'data mode' described above.

PATSy is also gaining emerging roles in the area of modelling – both as a source of data for models of language production (for example) and as a 'level playing field' for evaluating competing models.

Studying clinical reasoning with PATSy

PATSy was used in an investigation of clinical reasoning by speech and language pathology students (Cox and Lum, 2003). Students used PATSy in a cognitive neuropsychology course in aphasia. The course adopted an information-processing approach to normal and pathological language production.

The task of diagnosis is relatively ill-structured and requires a large amount of domain knowledge. Often there are no 'prototypical' cases to guide the novice and a considerable amount of prior knowledge is required.

Test data on PATSy are interpretable at various levels of granularity (item-by-item, overall test scores, error patterns). The absolute scores and the error patterns are both of theoretical significance. Interpretation (at least in experts) may also be moderated by more global factors such as the 'severity' of the patient's condition and/or the patient's social and educational background. Confronted with a large menu of tests, students must plan and adopt an orderly approach to their enquiries. They must be capable of isolating and controlling particular factors and must recognize that some factors may be confounded with others.

The nature of clinical reasoning expertise

The acquisition of clinical reasoning skills therefore imposes an enormous cognitive load on students and entails a large range of speech and language therapy-specific (SLT) and general reasoning (G) skills, including:

- extensive knowledge of the information-processing model of language comprehension and production (SLT)
- fluent knowledge of a wide range of neuropsychological tests – their purpose and format, together with an ability to quickly identify tests by name in terms of input/output modalities employed and aspects of cognition that they test (SLT)
- an ability to think of tests in abstract terms (i.e. a description language level mental representation) rather than assuming a test can measure only what its title implies that it can measure (G)
- an ability to think of patient performance in terms of a degraded normal model – this involves considerations of modalities of information processing (auditory, visual) and also level (input, central or output processing) (SLT)
- an ability to select the right level or granularity of information in a test, i.e. phoneme, word or sentence for a particular test of patient functioning (SLT)
- vigilance for particular error patterns and awareness of relevant pyscholinguistic parameters of verbal stimuli, e.g. spotting a patient's tendency to fail on words low in imageability or words that have low frequency of occurrence (G)
- general psychometric knowledge – in order to avoid simplistic interpretations or misinterpretations of errors made by the patient (G)
- hypothesis generation – an ability to focus on a question derived from theory (G)

- an ability to judge the extent to which evidence supports a hypothesis (G)
- deductive reasoning ability (as opposed to inductive 'template matching' and score profiling) (G).

As expertise develops, knowledge becomes increasingly compiled, automatic and implicit. Experts are often poor in communicating their expertise. For this reason, 'knowledge elicitation' methods have been developed by knowledge engineers in order to extract and (re)represent expert knowledge in artificial systems. Lyon et al. (1992) point out:

> Too often the teacher is unable to make clear and explicit to the medical student the path his or her mind has taken in diagnostic decision making ... there is an ever-growing discrepency between the continuously increasing multitude of facts and the low level of understanding of how to use them.

Calls for professional educators to externalize and make explicit their clinical reasoning (to 'model critical thinking') in teaching have been made (Facione and Facione, 1996). Munroe (1996) identified the use of 'coded meanings' or 'encryption' as a major barrier to the clear articulation of reasoning by occupational therapists to their students. This coding was found to take the form of commonly used and personal adages, e.g. 'keeping the door open', 'keeping the client in the picture'. Munroe (1996) does not suggest that students interpret such adages literally, but that students have difficulty appreciating the full richness, diversity and complexity of the clinician's underlying meaning.

Biases of various kinds also abound in clinical reasoning, as they do in 'everyday' thinking. These include a tendency to overconfidence resulting from the overemphasis of positive test findings and the downplaying of negative ones (Lyon et al., 1992). Using simulated medical diagnosis tasks, McKenzie (1997) has demonstrated a tendency of subjects to underweight evidence for alternative hypotheses and that this is a sufficient condition for the development of overconfidence in evidence for the subject's focal hypothesis. Other common reasoning biases include base-rate and 'gamblers' fallacies (e.g. Robertson, 1999).

Such biases are difficult to override instructionally and must be taken into account in the design of professional education programmes. It has been shown that the training of abstract principles (rules of logic) is much more effective when the rules are illustrated with examples that 'fit' with students' preconceptions; for example, problem solving with a real-life situation compared to manipulating abstract symbols. Such preconceptions include societal rules or 'permissions schemas', such as 'consumers of alchohol must be over 18' as opposed to abstract representations such as 'given "if P then Q" and observing not-Q, what follows?' (Cheng et al., 1986).

Three factors have been argued to account for clinicians' diagnostic skill (Lyon et al., 1992):

- experience, which results in the distillation of increasingly abstract cognitive constructs
- induction or pattern recognition (e.g. seeing trends, syndromes, etc., in sets of test scores)
- hypothetico-deductive reasoning (i.e. systematic generation and testing of hypotheses derived from theory or models).

Which of the factors is more important is still a source of debate, despite extensive clinical reasoning research. Parallel debates are taking place in the domain of education, especially science education. Can 'rules for reasoning' be taught? Are they effective? Is it better to teach them in domain-specific contexts across the curriculum, or separately in the form of domain-independent 'critical thinking' courses? Lum (2002), in her book *Scientific Thinking in Speech and Language Therapy*, opts to model critical thinking with examples drawn from speech and language therapy practice. Other authors have chosen domain-independent approaches (Nisbett, 1993; Halpern, 1996; Marzano et al., 1988).

A recent review of experts' and novices' differences in diagnostic reasoning is provided by Cuthbert et al. (1999). Some of the ways in which expert diagnosis can be differentiated from that of trainees include:

- the selection of more relevant and critical cues from a case history
- better organization of domain knowledge
- longer chains of reasoning.

Novices lack experience and possess a limited number of (mentally) stored cases. Compared to experts, a novice's attempts at induction (which is a naturalistic mode of reasoning) will be unproductive. Hence the education of trainees should include training which aims to: (a) confine them (at least initially) to deductive rather than inductive modes of reasoning where the rules are explicit and theoretically driven, and (b) equip them with a rational structure for enquiring about unknown cases or disorders in the future. In the context of a case-based approach using PATSy, clinical placements, etc., they will, over time, also expand their case-base store to a point where induction can complement deduction productively. It must be stressed, however, that this transition to more heterogeneous modes cannot be rushed.

As the studies reviewed above indicate, most clinical reasoning work to date has been conducted in scientific and medical education contexts, with some activity in occupational therapy (reflected in two special issues of the *British Journal of Occupational Therapy*; e.g. Lyon et al., 1992). However, few if any formal studies of clinical reasoning in speech and language therapy have been conducted to date.

An SLT study of student reasoning using PATSy

The aims of the study (Cox and Lum, 2003) were to investigate questions such as: 'How does the clinical reasoning of better students differ from that of poorer students?' and 'What implications might the results have for improving the design of SLT educational programmes?' Another aim was to test a prediction, from the literature on expertise, that better students would outperform poorer students in terms of both general reasoning skills and speech and language therapy-specific knowledge. Thirty-eight third-year speech and language therapy students participated in the study. Of these, three students were excluded due to failure to complete the pre- and post-tests and (in one case) personal difficulties that interfered with performance.

PATSy was closely integrated into a cognitive neuropsychology course on acquired language disorders. Students were referred to numerous PATSy cases in lectures during the semester and were expected to use PATSy as a course requirement. Participants were also pre-tested on a range of general and speech and language therapy-specific tests of knowledge and reasoning.

The general reasoning pre-tests included the Broadbent and Berry (1987) 'River pollution' computer-based task in which the goal is to diagnose which of 16 factories is responsible for polluting a river by performing chemical tests efficiently. This task yielded three scores for each subject – number of chemical tests performed to identify polluter, number of attempts required to identify the guilty factory, time taken to solution. This task was chosen as it seems to require search heuristics of a kind also required in clinical diagnosis.

The well-known Wason (1966) four-card deductive reasoning task was also used as a general reasoning pre-test, together with a Graduate Record Examination (GRE) test. In the Wason task, a row of four cards is presented. The cards are labelled 'A', 'K', '4' and '7'. Subjects are informed of the rule 'If there is a vowel on one side of the card, then there is an even number on the other side of the card'. They are asked 'What card or cards do you have to turn over to test the rule?' Two versions were used, the original 'abstract' version described above, and an equivalent 'realistic' version based on the rule 'If a person is drinking beer, then the person must be over 18 years old'. These versions were scored in a manner that yielded a score range of -2 to $+2$.

The GRE test consisted of two types of item – analytical reasoning puzzles (constraint-satisfaction problems) and verbal reasoning items. GRE items have a multiple-choice response format and pose problems which often entail constraint-satisfaction reasoning (e.g. assigning people to offices under various constraints such as who smokes or not, adjacency requirements, a particular person to be assigned the room with a large window, etc.; see Cox and Brna (1995) for further details about this kind of test).

Two pre-tests of SLT-specific knowledge were also used. The first was a 'Test of test knowledge' (TOT) (developed by Dr Julie Morris at the University of Newcastle) and the second was a test of knowledge of the IP model (TOM). Sample TOT items are shown in Table 8.2.

Table 8.2 Sample items from the 'Test of test knowledge'.

The ADA minimal pairs test tests:	In the ADA minimal pairs test, the person:
(a) semantics	(a) sees two written stimuli
(b) phonological discrimination	(b) hears two rhyming words
(c) hearing	(c) hears two words or non-words
(d) word recognition	(d) hears two phonemes

The TOM test required participants to draw a 'box and arrow' diagram of the Patterson and Shewell (1987) model of language processing.

The diagrams were scored in terms of the number of correct components (maximum score 20). The TOT and TOM were administered on day 1 of the course and at the end of the semester. Another source of data consisted of detailed records of students' use of PATSy during the semester-long course (recorded via the system's logging facility). The students conducted a diagnosis of a previously unseen case on PATSy (DBL – a case of 'word-finding' difficulties in speech production) at the end of the semester. They used PATSy in examination mode and the system logged the tests which were 'administered' to DBL by each student. These records were similar to the one shown in Figure 8.7.

The main outcome measure for the study was students' marks on a 2000-word written assignment based on the PATSy exam case. The assignment required students to analyse and interpret the data from the unseen case and to give an account of his speech-production problems in accordance with a cognitive neuropsychological perspective. A major component of the assignment mark was based on the lecturer's assessment of how well the student presented arguments couched within a cognitive neuropsychological perspective. Argumentation and comprehensive consideration of relevant cognitive subsystems were positively weighted in marking. The students also underwent a repeat administration of the TOT and TOM tests.

Test description language (TDL)

To interpret the user–PATSy interaction protocols for the assessment case (DBL), a more abstract representation of tests in the form of a 'test description language' (TDL) was devised. This is because differently named tests can be similar in terms of the cognitive processes that they measure (Howard and Franklin 100 picture reading test and the ADA L2Wr reading-of-words test, for example). TDL representation also makes students' reasoning patterns more salient (Table 8.3). The TDL metadata tagging of test information in PATSy is in the process of being extended to allow PATSy content to be searched in more detail – in terms of the 'level' of a test (sub-word, word, sentence), for example. The TDL represents a test in terms of the cognitive modalities it assesses and the mode of response required from the patient. An example of the scheme in use is shown in in Table 8.3 – the TROG (Figure 8.9) is coded APSSy(Pt). Detailed analyses of the students' log data are presented in Cox and Lum (2003).

Two subgroups of student were identified on the basis of assignment marks – better scoring (equal or above median assignment mark) and poorer scoring (lower than median). The groups consisted of 15 'low' and 20 'high' students and the median assignment mark for all students was 15 (range 0–25).

Speech and language therapy-specific knowledge

On the test of test knowledge, both groups of students performed equally well at post-test, although poorer students started off with lower and more variable scores at the beginning of semester pre-test. Both groups showed equally poor knowledge of the IP model at pre-test, although by the end of the course they had improved considerably. Students who went on to do well on the assignment showed greater improvement in their knowledge of the IP model.

Table 8.3 Examples of TDL representations of subjects' testing sequence for case DBL in the course of diagnosis. Participants S6, S10 and S30 were third-year speech and language therapy students (NB shorter-than-average student test sequence examples chosen to save space – mean test sequence length for students = 20.6, s.d. = 9.2). Key to coding scheme: capital letters indicate stimulus modality(ies) of test; letter in parentheses indicates mode in which patient responds. Test stimulus modality codes: A = auditory, V = visual (e.g. written word), P = picture, S = semantic, Sy = syntax. Patient response modalities (in brackets): In = indicate (e.g. raise finger), Sp = spoken, Pt = point.

Subjects	S6		S10		S30	
Sequence	TDL	Test	TDL	Test	TDL	Test
1	AMPSSy(Pt)	TROG	AMPSSy(Pt)	TROG	A(In)	ADA L1
2	A(In)	ADA L1	A(Sp)	ADA R	AMPSSy(Pt)	TROG
3	A(In)	ADA P1	A(In)	ADA L1	A(In)	ADA P1
4	PS(Pt)	P&P Trees PP	V(In)	ADA L1Wr	A(In)	ADA P2
5	AS(In)	PALPA 49	V(Sp)	ADA RWr	A(In)	ADA L1
6	A(Sp)	ADA R	V(Sp)	ADA L2Wr	AS(In)	PALPA 49
7	SP(Sp)	H&Fl00 PN	VPS(Pt)	P&P Trees PW	PS(Pt)	P&P Tree PP
8	V(In)	ADA L1WR	PS(Pt)	P&P Trees PP	V(Sp)	ADA RWr
9			SP(Sp)	H&F 100 PN	A(Sp)	ADA R
10			VM(In)	STM MS vis	V(Sp)	ADA L2Wr
11			VM(Sp)	ST digit rec	V(Sp)	ADA RWr
12			AM(In)	STM MS aud	V(Sp)	H&F 100 Rdg
13					V(In)	ADA L1Wr

General reasoning

Students who performed above the median on the assignment also tended to perform better on the river pollution task. They demonstrated more efficient search strategies in the course of identifying the guilty factory (i.e. fewer chemical tests administered), as well as faster times to solution.

The GRE test results showed a different pattern, however. Students who did less well on the assignment tended to perform better on the GRE than students whose assignment scores were above the median. The higher GRE (analytical reasoning) scores observed in students scoring below the median on the assignment was interesting. Clearly, the students who did less well on the assignment were not intellectually lacking. One conclusion would seem to be that constraint-satisfaction puzzle solving is a skill that can be orthogonal to those required in diagnostic reasoning. Analytical reasoning problems are generally of the constraint-satisfaction puzzle variety in which there are a few, well-defined dimensions (six people to be assigned to six offices, for example) and well-defined constraints (one person must have the room with the large window, two are noisy, one needs quiet, etc.). Clinical reasoning is much more complex, ill-structured and varied in terms of the modes of reasoning required. Another possibility is that students who did less well on the written essay assignment perform better when given multiple choice response formats (as in the GRE) and vice versa.

Wason deductive reasoning performance was not correlated with assignment performance. Performance on the abstract version of the Wason four-card task by students was very similar to that typically reported in the literature (e.g. Wason, 1966; Cheng and Holyoak, 1985). On the abstract version of the task, no student made the logically correct card selection (fewer than 10% typically do so in reported studies), and 'affirming the consequent' (selection of card 'A' and card '4' instead of the correct response 'A' and '7') was the pattern shown by 68% of subjects. This represents a tendency to seek confirmation of a rule rather than disconfirming evidence, i.e. a 'confirmation bias'. In contrast, 66% of students chose the logically correct cards on a 'realistic' (age rule and alchohol drinking) version of the task, showing the usual dramatic effect of making the rule context more 'concrete' (Cheng and Holyoak, 1985).

Of the three kinds of domain-independent test (constraint-satisfaction/analytical reasoning, deductive reasoning and heuristic search), only performance on the river pollution (heuristic search) exercise correlated with assignment mark.

The failure of the Wason tasks to differentiate between better and poorer students in terms of assignment marks may have been because 'rule affirmation', rather than 'rule disconfirmation', tends to underlie the type of conditional reasoning practised clinically. Clinicians tend to reason validly about what follows when an antecedent condition is true (if P then Q), but, like most people, they reason much less validly when asked for valid conclusions given 'not q' ('not p' is a valid conclusion given 'not q').

Experience with PATSy

The results suggested that online interactions with the PATSy system during the semester were positively associated with end-of-term assignment scores. Specifically, 70% of students scoring above the median on the essay assignment had seen between four and six cases on PATSy during the semester. In contrast, only 53% of students scoring below the median had done so. Further analyses (Cox and Lum, 2003) suggested that the number of cases seen on PATSy during the semester was (positively) associated with students' exam performance to a greater extent than it was with essay assignment performance. Compared to the exam, the assignment required more knowledge of hypothesis testing and knowledge of a theoretical model of language processing.

Clinical reasoning study – discussion

The prediction that skilled clinical reasoning requires both domain-specific and domain-independent knowledge was supported to some extent. Efficient search heuristics and good knowledge of the IP model seem to be particularly important and there are implications of the results for student training. Students usually receive direct instruction on language processing theory but do not receive training in search heuristics – a key component of diagnostic reasoning. An interesting question, therefore, concerns the extent to which training on simulations such as the river pollution task might improve students' ability to apply useful strategies for efficiently 'homing in' on solutions. If improvements transferred to diagnostic reasoning contexts then there may be a case for the introduction of such domain-general skills training into health science curricula.

Conclusion

PATSy is an online, interactive multimedia case database for educators, clinicians and researchers. The system has been developed to provide students, clinicians and researchers with 'on-demand' access to people with speech and language disorders for pre- and in-service clinical training. Interactive learning environments such as PATSy offer numerous benefits, including unlimited opportunity for rehearsing skills such as diagnostic reasoning and test administration – a 'flight simulator' for speech and language therapy seems like a somewhat apt analogy.

PATSy provides an interactive environment in which students can be supported during the difficult transition from novice (mainly deductive) to expert (more heterogeneous) modes of reasoning. Interaction with cases on PATSy allows students to develop rule-based, deductive approaches to test selection, at the same time preventing cognitive overload and permitting repetition and rehearsal.

PATSy is also proving to be useful as a tool for collecting data on student reasoning and as a source of data and dissemination for researchers. The ethos of PATSy is that of a shared resource which is used, maintained and contributed to by members of the speech and language therapy community and other clinical and research communities. Further information is available on the website at www.patsy.ac.uk, including access to password-free 'walkthroughs' of the system. Interested readers are encouraged to contact the authors if they would like to be issued with a guest account.

Acknowledgements

The support of the Nuffield Foundation is gratefully acknowledged. Many thanks to Jonathan Kilgour for PATSy system programming, and for programming a computer version of the river pollution task. Thanks too to Dr Julie Morris for development of the test knowledge test, and to the third-year speech and language therapy students who participated in the clinical reasoning study.

References

Barrows HS (1985) How to Design a Problem-based Curriculum for the Pre-clinical Years. New York: Springer.

Bishop D (1989) TROG: Test of Reception of Grammar. University of Manchester: Department of Psychology.

Broadbent DE, Berry DC (1987) Explanation and verbalization in a computer-assisted search task. Quarterly Journal of Experimental Psychology 39A: 585–609.

Cheng PW, Holyoak KJ (1985) Pragmatic reasoning schemas. Cognitive Psychology 17: 391–416.

Cheng PW, Holyoak KJ, Nisbett RE, Oliver LM (1986) Pragmatic versus syntactic approaches to training deductive reasoning. Cognitive Psychology 18: 293–328.

Cox R, Brna P (1995) Supporting the use of external representations in problem solving: the need for flexible learning environments. Journal of Artificial Intelligence in Education 6: 239–302.

Cox R, Lum C (2003) The rôles of domain-specific and domain-independent knowledge in diagnostic reasoning: an investigation using PATSy (in preparation).

Cuthbert L, du Boulay B, Teather D, Teather B, Sharples M, du Boulay G (1999) Expert/novice differences in diagnosic medical cognition – a review of the literature. Cognitive Science Research Papers CSRP 508, School of Cognitive & Computing Sciences, University of Sussex.

Edelson DC (1996) Learning from cases and questions: the Socratic case-based teaching architecture. Journal of the Learning Sciences 5: 357–410.

Ellis AW, Young AW (1996) Human Cognitive Neuropsychology. Hove, UK: Psychology Press.

Facione NC, Facione PA (1996) Externalizing the critical thinking in knowledge development and clinical judgement. Nursing Outlook 44: 129–135.

Halpern DF (1996) Thought and Knowledge: An Introduction to Critical Thinking. Mahwah, NJ: Lawrence Erlbaum.

Hmelo CE (1995) Problem based learning: development of knowledge and reasoning strategies. Proceedings of the Seventeenth Annual Conference of the Cognitive Science Society. Hillsdale, NJ: Lawrence Erlbaum Associates, pp. 403–408.

Irby DM (1994) Three exemplary models of case-based teaching. Academic Medicine 69: 947–953.

Jonassen DH (1996) Scaffolding diagnostic reasoning in case-based learning environments. Journal of Computing in Higher Education 8: 48–68.

Kolodner JL (1993) Case-based reasoning. San Mateo, CA: Morgan Kaufmann.

Lum C (2002) Scientific Thinking in Speech and Language Therapy. Mahwah, NJ: Lawrence Erlbaum Associates.

Lum C, Cox R (1998) PATSy – a distributed multimedia assessment training system. International Journal of Communication Disorders 33: 170–175.

Lum C, Cox R, Kilgour J, Morris J, Tobin R (1999) PATSy: a multimedia Web-based resource for aphasiologists and neuropsychologists in research and education. Aphasiology 13: 573–579.

Lum C, Ellis A (1999) Why do some aphasics show an advantage on some tests of nonpropositional (automatic) speech? Brain & Language 70: 95–118.

Lyon HC, Healy JC, Bell JR, O'Donnell JF, Shultz EK, Moore-West M, Wigton RS, Hirai F, Beck JR (1992) PlanAlyzer, an interactive computer-assisted program to teach clinical problem solving in diagnosing anemia and coronary heart disease. Academic Medicine 67: 821–828.

McKenzie CRM (1997) Underweighting alternatives and overconfidence. Organizational Behavior and Human Decision Processes 71: 141–160.

Marzano RJ, Brandt RS, Hughes CS, Jones BF et al. (1988) Dimensions of Thinking: A Framework for Curriculum and Instruction. Alexandria, VA: Association for Supervision and Curriculum Development.

Munroe H (1996) Clinical reasoning in community occupational therapy. British Journal of Occupational Therapy 59: 196–202.

Nisbett RE (1993) Rules for Reasoning. Hillsdale, NJ: Lawrence Erlbaum Associates.

Patterson K, Shewell C (1987) Speak and spell: dissociations and word-class effects. In Coltheart M, Sartori G, Job R (eds) The Cognitive Neuropsychology of Language. Hillsdale, NJ: Lawrence Erlbaum Associates.

Riesbeck CK, Schank RC (1991) From training to teaching: techniques for case-base intelligent tutoring systems. In Burns H, Parlett JW, Luckhardt-Redfield C (eds) Intelligent Tutoring Systems: Evolutions in Design. Hillsdale, NJ: Lawrence Erlbaum Associates, pp. 177–193.

Robertson SI (1999) Types of Thinking. London: Routledge.

Schank RC (1991) Case-based Teaching: Four Experiences in Educational Software Design (Technical Report No. 7). Chicago, IL: Northwestern University, The Institute for the Learning Sciences.

Stackhouse J, Wells WC (1997) Children's Speech and Literacy: A Psycholinguistic Framework. London: Whurr.

Wason PC (1966) Reasoning. In Foss B (ed.) New Horizons in Psychology. Harmondsworth: Penguin, pp. 135–151.

Williams SM (1993) Putting case-based learning into context: examples from legal, business and medical education. Journal of the Learning Sciences 2: 367–427.

Index

744180